Thorsons Introductory Guide to
THE ALEXANDER TECHNIQUE

D0339021

Other Thorsons Introductory Guides:

Acupuncture
Chiropractic
Healing
Herbalism
Homoeopathy
Hypnotherapy
Iridology
Kinesiology
Osteopathy
Reflexology
Shiatsu

By the same author:

Body Know-How: A practical guide to the use of the Alexander Technique in everyday life

Thorsons Introductory Guide to
THE ALEXANDER TECHNIQUE

Jonathan Drake

Thorsons
An Imprint of HarperCollins*Publishers*

Thorsons
An Imprint of HarperCollins*Publishers*
77–85 Fulham Palace Road,
Hammersmith, London W6 8JB

Published by Thorsons 1993
1 3 5 7 9 10 8 6 4 2

A catalogue record for this book
is available from the British Library

ISBN 0 7225 2779 9

Typeset by Harper Phototypesetters Limited,
Northampton, England
Printed in Great Britain by
The Guernsey Press Co. Ltd, Guernsey, Channel Islands

Contents

Acknowledgements

Many thanks to my editors at Thorsons, Sarah Sutton and Barbara Vesey. I am also very grateful to my colleagues: Alice Knight, who made many useful suggestions; John Naylor, who tempered Chapters 5 and 6; and Mervyn Waldman and Katia Cedar, who also commented on these chapters. Eddie Sellens and Bill and Olwen Cooter greatly improved readability. My wife Angela helped keep me on track throughout in many ways and provided the illustrations. These kind reviewers are not, of course, responsible for any errors I may have made, nor for the opinions expressed in this guide.

Introduction

The aim of this guide is to give you clear answers to your questions about the Alexander Technique: what it is, how it works, whom it can help with what kinds of problems and how to go about learning it.

The Alexander Technique is a method for recovering the grace and co-ordination that young children acquire naturally in the course of their development and which is largely lost by adulthood. It can help manage the stresses and strains of daily life, whether this involves coping with household tasks, sitting at a computer or refining the most demanding of skills, such as playing a musical instrument. No other method of stress management, to my knowledge, tackles the essential link between mind and body as you come into contact with a stressful stimulus. At that moment you need a certain amount of tension in the right parts of your body to function at your best. Getting uptight and, sometime later, trying to relax or to unwind through vigorous exercise is not satisfactory. Not only may you be failing to meet the challenges of your stressful life, but you may be undermining your health through your attempts to escape from stress. This is often regarded as 'living life to the full'!

Apart from its preventive aspects, most people are drawn to the Alexander Technique because it can be a vital tool in the process of recovery from ill-health. Although it is often associated with alleviating back pain, this book explains how the Technique can help bring about improvement in a wide variety of health problems and many other areas of your life. Orthodox medicine and other therapies can never remedy completely the psychosomatic diseases that we may, unwittingly, be creating for ourselves.

'What am I doing to myself to cause my difficulties?' was the question F. M. Alexander asked over a hundred years ago. An actor, he had been troubled by increasing hoarseness. Doctors told him that there was no underlying physical problem with his vocal cords, and they were unable to tell him what might be doing to impair his voice. Rest only relieved his condition temporarily, so overdoing it was only part of the problem.

Determined to find a solution, he embarked on an extraordinarily thorough investigation. He used mirrors for self-observation and made various experiments on himself. He discovered – among other things – that his vocal trouble was but one consequence of misusing muscles throughout his body. He soon noticed that most people showed similar patterns of 'malcoordination'. Alexander's initial experimentation spanned nine years, during which time he pioneered a method to improve what he called the 'use of self' and he restored his voice completely.

Alexander's technique encourages us to be mindful of a crucial aspect of our co-ordination – the dynamic relationship between head, neck and torso – that influences most of our functioning.

Not that it is easy to help ourselves – much as we may wish to do so. We are all creatures of habit. Our reactions and patterns of movement and posture are deeply entrenched. *We* are the problem and it is only by revolutionizing our understanding of ourselves that we can hope to make worthwhile change in our lives.

While the Alexander Technique is a method of self-help, the role of a teacher is vital at the beginning and often at other stages in the learning process, as you will see. What individual lessons involve and how to choose a competent teacher are described in Chapter 5.

A neglected area – covered in Chapter 6 – is the question of how the Technique compares with other educational and therapeutic approaches. Are there any conflicts? Is the Technique a cure-all? It can come perilously close to sounding like one, but no single system holds all the answers. None the less, as you will see, the Technique is a powerful catalyst for change and for enhancing health and well-being. I cannot think of one area of my life that has not been enriched by my understanding of the Technique.

I hope the possibilities of the Alexander Technique outlined in this book will encourage you to investigate further and perhaps take lessons.

Note: To avoid the clumsiness of he/she, etc., I have used he/him/his throughout to refer to either gender, unless the context indicates otherwise.

Chapter 1

What the Alexander Technique Is and How It Can Help

Strictly speaking, the Alexander Technique should not be lumped together with *any* therapeutic method, orthodox or alternative. It is first and foremost to do with *self-discovery and re-education.* Its brief is simple: *How well am I using myself – my mind/body – in all my daily activities?*

You might like to try these simple tests. Can you:

1. turn your head freely on your neck to the sides without turning your shoulders? (Don't cheat by tightening your shoulders!)
2. open your mouth wide without pulling back your head or tucking in your chin?
3. raise your arms above your head without tightening and arching your lower back?
4. go into a squat without lifting your heels from the ground – with ease?

If you cannot answer an unequivocal 'yes' to all these, your co-ordination is not what it should be!

How much improvement can you expect? You will only really know after you have experienced the difference that Alexander lessons make: movements that were previously jerky, tense and laborious become, with the help of a teacher's hands, smoother, lighter, freer and easier. This change, which affects the whole body and comes about through a radical redistribution of muscle tone, is often profoundly healing. You feel more at one with yourself, less a bundle of disconnected or disowned parts.

After a basic course of lessons you will have learned how to maintain this improved body use and perhaps make further progress on your own. This empowers you to be much more responsible for your own health and well-being.

Why 'Good' Posture Is Bad for You

'Posture' implies something fixed and static – how to hold yourself 'correctly' in a certain position. What is called posture is only a 'freeze-frame' of a continuous process of movement.

All of us have an idea about what constitutes 'good' posture: holding ourselves 'upright', shoulders back, chin in, stomach in, tail tucked in and so on. And the harder we try, the stiffer we become! Yet it is a very common belief that if only we tried a little harder, or learned to relax more, or did the right exercises, we could improve our posture. Wrong! At best we just shift the problem around; at worst we create more problems than we may have already.

You might like to try another little experiment: see if you can remain completely still. Apart from your breathing movements and the pulsing of blood through your body, you will notice a very slight wavering, rocking movement taking place continually as your body maintains its balance. Physiologists tell us that at the microscopic level there is a constantly changing pattern of activation of millions of tiny muscle fibres; as parts of muscle relax, other parts work to maintain our overall balance of muscle tone. Staying still for any length of time makes you experience an almost irresistible urge to fidget. The lesson here? Posture has a dynamic quality: it involves change and balance at many levels of the organism.

In fact there is a pattern of body use operating at all times. Adjusting one part of the body has repercussions for the whole system. We are more than the sum of our physical parts. We are each a *mind/body*, an interacting system of mental and physical processes.

USE AFFECTS FUNCTIONING

In Chapter 2 you will learn about the remarkable F. Matthias Alexander. His Technique emerged from his conclusion that the problems affecting his voice were symptoms of a general 'malcoordination'; he also discovered that a vital part of the solution lay in changing his mental approach.

When he began teaching other actors what he had learned they would frequently report to him that – just as he himself had experienced – as their co-ordination improved, so did a whole host of health problems. Alexander deduced, therefore, that *use has a profound influence on functioning*. His teaching experience over the next 60 years, and that of succeeding generations of teachers, bears out the thesis that malcoordination is a prominent factor in many chronic conditions.

So just how common is malcoordination, or *misuse*, as Alexander called it? Dr Barlow, a consultant in physical medicine and teacher of the Alexander Technique, conducted research assessing the posture of groups of students starting physical education and performing arts courses. [1] He was forced to conclude that over 80 per cent showed substantial or severe postural defects which *worsened* if they followed the remedial exercises prescribed. Only those receiving Alexander lessons showed significant improvement.

WHY WE GO WRONG

If misuse is so prevalent, where does it start? Young children have an alertness and poise that allow them to move freely and easily without strain. Within a few months – remarkable when you consider the comparative size and weight of their heads – infants have sufficient neck and head control to sit unsupported. Walking is achieved at approximately one year old without, of course, any *conscious* effort. Children possess tremendous natural will and energy to explore their surroundings and experiment with new patterns of movement. Learning takes place on a subconscious level and at an incredible rate. However, as children get older, certain habits develop as a result of 'the trials of life' that interfere with this natural co-ordination and functioning.

At school, children spend a lot of time sitting, often on chairs

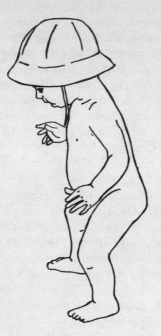

Figure 1: This eight-month-old infant already displays a supple, powerful and co-ordinated use of his legs

and at tables that are not appropriate heights. Nowadays there is little instruction in the art of holding pens and pencils to minimize tension in the writing arm as well as in the neck and other parts of the body. Also, most children learn about body use by imitating parents and teachers, who are not usually – even with the best of intentions – very good role models. A child's personality is also forming, and this produces changes in his posture and body language to reflect the architecture of his inner world. At the same time, most children want to please others; this striving for approval can result in physical as well as mental distortions.

Paul, in his forties, came for lessons suffering from chronic back pain made worse on walking any distance. He suddenly remembered, in the course of a lesson, that when he was a few years old he used to try to walk like his father. 'He walked with a slight sway to one side, and that's just what I'm doing now!' Over the course of the next few lessons, Paul's walking improved dramatically and his back pain began to ease.

In addition, much of what passes for 'physical education' removes a little more of children's natural poise. Most forms of fitness training and many specialized activities such as gymnastics, ballet and hockey can severely compromise good body use. Competitive sport – for the few who excel – can be a source of great pleasure and pride – but for how long? For the rest of us it can be a turn-off for life: by adulthood, if not before, most physical activity comes to be seen as a chore and sport becomes something we watch on TV.

To the adolescent, trying to cope with rapid physical and mental changes and reacting to peer and other social pressures, style and body language become very important. The 'casual', slumped look – if not already the norm – almost invariably becomes the predominant mode of body use.

Women, too, face particular stresses. There are all sorts of expectations, fostered by the fashion industry, about what women should be wearing. Tight skirts and jeans and high-heeled shoes limit good body use. The challenge of childbearing is frequently 'the straw that breaks the camel's back'. A new baby brings sleepless nights, 'mother's hip' (thrusting one hip out to perch the baby on) and perhaps the stresses of work both in and outside the home with little opportunity for rest and recuperation (not to mention the demands that other family members may make).

The Alexander Technique has an important role in facilitating a more natural birth.

Jean had a basic course of Alexander lessons some months before she became pregnant. As it turned out she had a particularly difficult and prolonged labour. But when asked whether the Technique had helped her during her pregnancy and afterwards she said she had really noticed how badly most women in the antenatal classes stood and moved about. She had felt a great sense of ease and freedom even in the final stages of pregnancy. The greatest benefits, though, came postnatally: 'I found myself being able to do all the things a mother has to do without strain, coping well and being able to return to work without worrying that my old back problem was going to recur.'

For many people, work involves static positions and repetitive activities, far removed from the hunter-gatherer lifestyle of our distant ancestors (although people who have physically demanding jobs – gardeners, farmers and nurses, for example – are not immune to back problems: on the contrary). Strenuous attempts to compensate for the shortcomings of our daily round – working out in a gym, jogging, etc. – may actually do more harm than good because we are more likely to consolidate the very patterns of misuse we would like to be free of.

Finally, accidents and injuries, the 'fall-out' of certain illnesses and prolonged periods of inactivity while convalescing – can all leave their mark on posture and body use.

Given this litany of possible difficulties, it is hardly surprising that Barlow found less than 5 per cent of the students he surveyed to be relatively free from postural defects.

The Health Benefits

What do you value in your life? What do you want to achieve? Some people make health more important than anything else. It is arguable that this is a worthy end in itself, but whatever your aspirations might be, health is an important *means* to those ends. And one of the most neglected factors influencing health – over which you have a large degree of control – is how effectively and efficiently you *use* yourself in your daily activities.

This has both preventive and remedial aspects and is still largely ignored by most doctors and health professionals. If a doctor takes a predominantly fatalistic view of health or narrows his concern to prosaic health education messages – to do with diet, moderate exercise and avoidance of harmful drugs (important though these messages are) – an opportunity to refer patients for help elsewhere is being missed. Alexander teachers not infrequently hear 'but my doctor told me that I would just have to learn to live with my backache.' But your mind/body has greater powers of recovery than that.

In 1937, 19 doctors co-signed a letter to the *British Medical Journal*: [2]

' . . .We have observed the beneficial changes in use and functioning which have been brought about by the employment of Alexander's technique in the patients we have sent to him for help – even in cases of so-called 'chronic disease' – while those of us who have been his pupils have personally experienced equally beneficial results. We are convinced that Alexander is justified in contending that ''an unsatisfactory manner of use, by interfering with general functioning, constitutes a predisposing cause of disorder and disease''; and that *diagnosis of a patient's troubles must remain incomplete* [unless] the influence of use upon functioning is taken into consideration.' [italics added]

These physicians went on to suggest that some knowledge of the Technique should perhaps be included in medical training, pending further investigation. Yet this letter prompted no such innovation in the standard medical curriculum.

Unfortunately even some alternative or complementary practitioners operate largely from the same assumptions as do most doctors. This situation will continue as long as patients are reluctant to take responsibility for their own health and well-being and, it has to be said (though it may sound cynical), as long as it serves the interests of doctors and therapists not to help patients to help themselves.

Alexander's four books and Dr Barlow's work contain many case histories in which improvement in body use was accompanied by the resolution of symptoms. The Alexander

Technique, therefore, has a significant role to play both in prevention and recovery. What follows is by no means an exhaustive list, but an indication of the *kinds* of conditions that can frequently be helped by the Technique:

• back and neck pain
• frozen shoulder
• tennis elbow
• repetitive strain disorders
• arthritis
• nerve/muscle/bone disorders
• stress-related, psychosomatic conditions: headaches, migraines, respiratory and gastro-intestinal problems, hyper-tension
• pregnancy/postnatal problems
• recovery from prolonged illness
• recovery after accidents, e.g. whiplash
• depression and anxiety states

Learning How to Learn

The Alexander Technique is essentially a 'pre-technique' which can be applied to improving the performance of all activities. It can help us clarify our thinking so that we can proceed in any endeavour in a less random, 'trial-and-error' way.

Have you ever felt awkward, clumsy and all tied up in knots while struggling with limited success to master a particular skill? I certainly have. Swimming, for instance, was always a source of discomfort for me. I could, at least, swim – but only after a fashion! My 'style' consisted of a very laboured breast stroke with my head held back high out of the water and tension gripping the whole of my body. Since applying the Technique I am now much more aware of how to eliminate unnecessary tension. I have been more able to let the water support me and to let the swimming 'do itself'. (For a fuller account of this see my book *Body Know-How*.)

If we get caught up in one aspect of a given activity, we can lose sight of the whole. Alexander underlined the fact that *concentration* – which we normally think of as a good thing – may be harmful if it produces unnecessary tension. It usually involves forcing our minds to focus on something that would not otherwise hold our attention; or it may be part of the struggle to be right – at all costs – producing great rigidity, physically and mentally.

POISE AND CONFIDENCE
How do you experience yourself? What attitude have you to your body? Some of us cut ourselves off from our physical being as much as we possibly can. Women in particular often have very negative attitudes to their appearance, worrying about whether they are the 'right' size or shape – but these concerns are affected by society's changing fashions and shifting medical goal posts. And it is all too easy to neglect the body until the eleventh hour when pain makes us give it some attention. Taking pain-killers only delays our having to face the reasons for our pain. For someone who is more conscious of himself in an ongoing way as a psycho-physical being, the body has its own intelligence. You can listen to it, take heed of its promptings and work with it. It can tell you much more about your needs than you might think.

If we regard our bodies merely as objects we run the risk of producing progressive strain through neglect. Many people slump at desks most of the day: the altered pressures in their bodies will produce severe disturbance of psychosomatic functioning sooner or later. If, on the other hand, we can learn to experience ourselves as sensitive instruments through which we live life, we will come to see the value of attending to *how* we carry out our daily activities.

Once you learn to live in harmony with your body and know what you can reasonably expect of it, when you know that in most circumstances you are using it well, your whole outlook on life will change. You will be less afraid of not coping and you will be more able to approach new challenges and opportunities with the knowledge and confidence that come with being more in command of yourself. Most of us once had these attractive qualities; they can, in large measure, be restored to us by the Alexander Technique.

THE PERFORMING ARTS

It is in the fields of drama, music and dance that the Alexander Technique has become most widely established. Alexander teachers work at all the major colleges of performing arts in London and in some other British and foreign cities. Performing artists need methods that work, so they look to the Alexander Technique to help them maximize their talents. It can help prevent and alleviate many of the vocal and repetitive strain problems as well as back pain and other injuries frequently suffered by performers. Of greater significance, perhaps, is the light it can bring to bear on the mental and physical preparation needed for an artist to give an optimal performance.

EVERYDAY LIFE

All of us can be creative in our daily lives and in our relationships with others. Possible – and certainly desirable – is what the Buddhists call *mindful awareness*: attention to detail, to the simple acts that make up daily life. We can cherish the incredible sensitivity and responsiveness of our psycho-physical selves. The Alexander Technique gives us special access to this world.

Chapter 2

The Key Principles
of the Technique

The beauty of the Alexander Technique – apart from the aesthetic of the properly co-ordinated movement it leads to – is the simplicity, clarity and power of its central ideas. These ideas arose from Alexander's practical experience, not from any theoretical speculation. They are, therefore, quite difficult to explain in words: they only carry real meaning once you have experienced them in lessons and start applying them in your life.

The Primary Control

The Alexander Technique is about developing an awareness of the basic patterns of our movements so that we may have more conscious control of ourselves in all our activities. The key to this is the head-neck-back relationship, or *primary control*.

Alexander used this expression to refer to the central organizing principle of our co-ordination (or lack of it). He discovered that the relationship between one's head, neck and back sets the tone for everything else: the relationship of all other body parts, ease of breathing – most aspects of functioning are directly or indirectly influenced by it.

He observed that there is an almost universal tendency, when *any* movement is initiated, to precede and accompany it with an increase in the level of tension in the muscles of the neck. This tension pulls the head back and down towards the shoulders and can be observed most clearly in the act of getting up from a seated position or sitting down – see Figure 2. You might like to try it: slow the movement down as much as you can and, if you touch the back of your neck, you will feel the large muscles

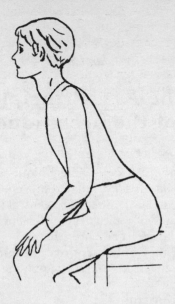

Figure 2: Standing up/sitting down is done at the cost of excessive
neck tension and postural distortion

tensing and your head pulling back – particularly as you first
move to sit down on or stand up from the chair.

Now, in an adult the head weighs roughly 10 lb (4 kg). If it
is not balanced easily on the top of the neck, the downward
pressure has serious consequences for the rest of the body. For
one thing, it puts considerable pressure on the joints all the way
down the spine. Fluid is squeezed out of the intervertebral discs
to such an extent that at the end of each day most of us are more
than half-an-inch (1.6 cm) shorter than we were at the start of
the day. (This loss, of course, is largely restored during rest.)
Every joint space in the body tends to be reduced by this
pressure – even to the tips of the toes and fingers.

Mary, in her late twenties, was booked in for an operation on her
knees, which had become increasingly painful and stiff. She worked

on an assembly line in the day. In her spare time she did virtually nothing except sport, sport, sport! – mostly football and squash. I asked her how she bent down to a low squash ball. It was immediately noticeable that she stiffened her neck, pressed downwards and her knees tended to pull in towards each other. She was advised to reduce her sporting activities drastically – at least for a while – which advice she chose to ignore, although she did learn to put less pressure on her joints while bending and to allow her knees to flex forward and slightly apart from each other over her feet. She remarked how odd it had felt at first but within a few weeks of Alexander lessons her symptoms improved dramatically and the operation was cancelled.

Excessive muscle tension will be used in some parts of the body to compensate for muscles that have become too slack elsewhere. This is what happens in the all-too-common standing posture seen nowadays – swayback – where there is a tendency to lean on the lower back. At least as serious a potential health risk as this pressure on the spine is the effect of altered body mechanics on the functioning of the internal organs. Pressures inside the chest, abdominal and pelvic cavities will be changed and the blood and nerve supplies to the internal organs will be affected. Over many years this cumulative disturbance of function can be serious and even life-threatening.

When the primary control functions as it should there is sufficient *release* in the neck muscles to allow the head to balance delicately at the top of the spine. Instead of the head inclining backwards and downwards under the force of gravity it is orientated in a forward and upward direction, producing a lengthening of the spine and a broadening of the torso.

The question is, how is this dynamic release to be achieved?

End-gaining

Alexander found that any *direct* attempt to hold his body in the position he thought was correct for reciting was counter-productive. At best he shifted the faulty tension elsewhere, producing other problems; at worst he made himself quite stiff and rigid. He used the term *end-gaining* to describe these tension-creating struggles towards attaining our goals. Even if we appear to succeed we may have created all sorts of unintended effects on the way – strains on certain parts of the body or so much fatigue that we may be unable to meet the next challenge. This relentless striving frequently leads to failure and disappointment; it wastes the energy we could be using to find more effective ways of accomplishing what we want to do.

NEVER UNDERESTIMATE HABIT

It is commonly believed that it is possible to put things right by *doing* the right thing. However, we are deluding ourselves if we think that patterns of movement can be changed simply by deciding to do them differently, by doing the right exercises or by 'relaxing' a little more. *We like to think we are free to do what we want, but the fact is that we invariably respond in habitual ways to familiar situations.* Of course this is necessary – to some degree; if every single action had to be worked out afresh, we would never make it out of bed in the morning!

The point is that our patterns should be our servants, not our masters. If we aspire to real change, we need to question in a fundamental way exactly *how* we go about our everyday activities. We will discover how little we actually *know* about what we are doing and how little control we have over our basic patterns of movement. All that needs changing cannot be changed at once – nor should we try. What we can do is to tackle small things first and be patient while the larger changes slowly come about. An extraordinary transformation can then take place: when people look back after a course of Alexander lessons, they are often surprised to see just how far they have travelled.

FAULTY BODY SENSE

All our movements are guided by our body sense, technically called *kinaesthesia* (*kin* = movement, *aesthesia* = sensation): that is, we 'feel out' how to move, either consciously or – more usually – subconsciously. There is no problem if our kinaesthesia is accurate. However, in most of us the kinaesthetic information is misinterpreted or does not reach our consciousness and then our posture, patterns of movement and co-ordination will be impaired. This disturbing fact becomes readily apparent on starting to learn the Alexander Technique: orientations in space such as up or down, forwards or backwards are frequently confused and the amount of tension required to carry out a particular movement is often grossly overestimated. Even lying down, it can be surprising to discover just how much you are still doing when you *feel* you are doing nothing!

So, closely linked to habit is doing what feels right and 'comfortable'. If, however, what feels right is actually *wrong*, then we will compound the problem if we rely mainly on the same mechanism, kinaesthesia (which would not be registering accurately) – to put us right. We should avoid trying to 'feel out' how to be right, according to Alexander, because it is bound to lead us astray. Instead we should aim to become more aware of – and therefore more able to *prevent* – what is wrong.

It follows, therefore, that *what is required will necessarily feel wrong, at first*! As one senior Alexander Technique teacher used to say, 'In time you will become less wrong; sometimes you may even be right!'

This essentially 'negative', indirect approach can be puzzling when first encountered. It goes against the grain. To put something right we want to know what we have to *do*. Alexander found that it was this 'doing' – which felt right and was in fact wrong – which had to be *un*done.

The question then arises: how do I know when I attempt to improve my pattern of body use whether what feels wrong is in fact right or is a 'different kind of badly'? To guide you between the devil and the deep blue sea, a teacher's help is indispensable.

Letting Yourself Be

The turning point in Alexander's search for a solution to his vocal trouble came when he realized that the only way he could change the bodily misuse he adopted when projecting his voice was to change his thinking. Up to that point he had assumed that his problem was basically a physical one. He eventually came to see that he only had to *think* of reciting and he would immediately begin stiffening his neck, pulling back his head and distorting his stature. Hence the importance of what Alexander called *inhibition*: the decision to stop or delay his response at the critical moment when he intended to recite. Thus were the chains linking the automatic response to a familiar stimulus to be weakened.

Non-doing is the physical aspect of this mental 'inhibition'. If you refuse to press ahead with your usual way of doing things – associated with the faulty pattern of use – then you can begin to 'let yourself be'. New and more economical ways of achieving your goals can then be found.

There is a popular association of the term 'inhibition' with repression, but this was not at all what Alexander meant. On the contrary, only by delaying his habitual response could he then make a more conscious and reasoned choice about whether to proceed in the usual manner, do nothing at all, or do something entirely different. He was interested in recovering *flexibility* of response, whether that response was predominantly physical or psychological. Thus inhibition and non-doing in fact allow for greater freedom; spontaneity and creativity are encouraged.

Putting a stop to your habitual response is the first step, but how is it possible to restore and maintain an improved relationship between your neck, head and back while carrying out any activity?

THE IMPORTANCE OF 'DIRECTIONS'

The answer lies in what Alexander called giving 'directions': a process of thinking – of projecting – the appropriate messages to the primary control rather than trying physically to put the head in a better orientation to the neck and torso. Since the body does not respond readily to negative messages, positive ones should be sent. And these directions are to be given in the proper order, with no attempt to *make* them happen. In time they will produce the necessary changes and all work together. I shall now try to describe – as best I can – what this entails, although it

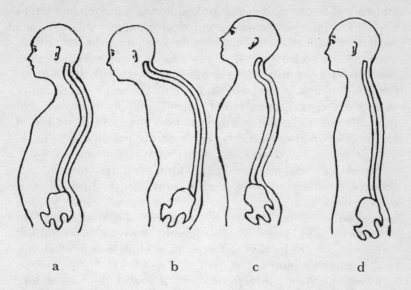

a   b   c   d

Figure 3: Styles of body use: central importance of the spine.
a) swayback; b) lumbar curve lost; c) 'military' posture;
d) condition of poise

is essentially something that has to be experienced to be understood.

The directions to the primary control are: *Let the neck be free* in order *to let the head go forward and up/out* in order *to let the spine lengthen and the torso widen*. *Neck free, head forward* results in a kind of 'unlocking' of the head on the neck. A helpful analogy – an example of Dr Barlow's – is to clench your fist and lock your wrist. When you release the clenched muscles of your fist you will notice that it rotates forward a little on your wrist; your hand is then free to move in any direction. In a similar way the 'unjamming' of your head involves an almost imperceptible forward rotation of your head on your neck. This releases your head so it can move in any way you want it to.

The next directions – immediately following 'Neck free,

head forward' – are *Let the head go up/out to let the spine lengthen and the torso widen*. Alexander lessons encourage a longer and wider back. A military-style posture produces an over-lengthened back not balanced by the appropriate widening; the lower back and neck are arched. What is very common nowadays, though, is a swayback posture where both length and width are lacking; the middle back is rounded and curves in the neck and lower back are also exaggerated. A further possibility is a back that is totally rounded, all length lost; here the normal neck and lower back curves are largely eradicated. (In practice these kinds of misuse are not always as distinct as I have described.)

The Alexander teacher aims to stimulate a dynamic balance between all these opposing tendencies within the body. This is done with a subtle use of his hands so that a more natural organization of body parts is achieved and maintained in movement. The pupil is also taught how to give himself directions so as to be able to co-ordinate himself well, when not in the teacher's hands.

These primary directions are followed by secondary directions to the arms and legs. At a later stage the pupil will be able to let more of these directions inform increasingly complicated patterns of movement. In this way a totally new pattern of movement is learned. This 'thinking in activity' tends to become more automatic in time; attention to all the details will not be so necessary and it becomes possible to focus on one aspect of a movement that needs attention while keeping a 'watching brief' on the whole pattern.

So, Alexander drew attention in a practical way to the unity of what we often think of as separate entities – our physical and psychological selves. Our intentions are inextricably expressed in our muscular responses. Unless we can loosen the bonds between stimulus and automatic response, our general standard of functioning will decline rapidly with each passing year.

Alexander urged us to pay more attention to the *means whereby* we may accomplish our ends. By becoming more cognizant of our attempts to cram more and more into life and the consequences of these attempts – increased emotional and

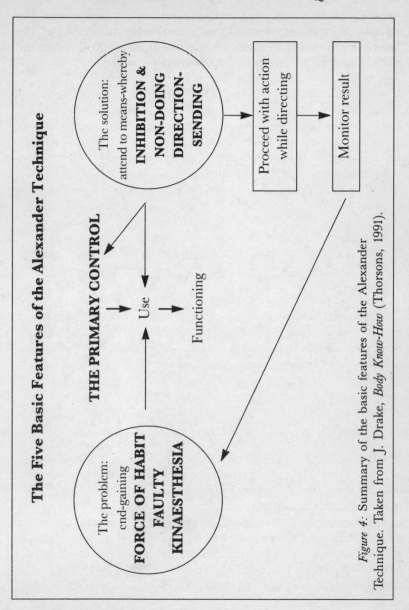

Figure 4: Summary of the basic features of the Alexander
Technique. Taken from J. Drake, *Body Know-How* (Thorsons, 1991).

physical tension – we can choose, in time, to compromise our well-being less and less. This requires hard work, but the rewards are great: an inner harmony, improved health and the satisfaction of reaching more of our aspirations.

Chapter 3

F. M. Alexander
The Man Behind the Technique

It's not easy to portray F. M. Alexander: there is no definitive biography[1] and little autobiographical material on which to draw. Judging by the accounts that do exist he seems to have been an extraordinary man, a pioneering genius who was single-minded in his commitment to 'the work'. Sketchy though the description that follows must be, it may satisfy some of your curiosity about him, how the Technique came into being and the course it has taken up to today.

Alexander's Early Days
Frederick Matthias Alexander was born in Tasmania in 1869. Despite an outdoor life with plenty of opportunities for boating, fishing, swimming and horse-riding he was rather sickly as a child, suffering frequently with respiratory and nasal infections. From an early age he was drawn to acting. Against the wishes of his father, who did not want his eldest son to be a 'strolling player and vagabond', 'FM' (as he liked to be called) decided to pursue a career as a reciter. To help pay for his professional training he took various part-time clerical and accountancy jobs.

He had made quite a name for himself as a reciter of humorous and dramatic pieces when he was increasingly troubled by the tendency of his voice to fail towards the end of recitals despite following, to the letter, medical advice to rest properly beforehand. At a particularly important engagement he could barely speak by the end of the evening and he contemplated giving up his stage career. He went back to his doctor, who could only suggest that he carry on with the treatment. This was unacceptable to Alexander, who posed the following, crucial question: 'Is it not fair, then, to conclude that it was something I was doing that evening in using my voice that was the cause of the trouble?' After reflecting for a moment, his doctor agreed that it must be so. 'Can you tell me then', Alexander asked him, 'what it was that I did that caused the trouble?' Since his doctor could give him no lead, Alexander resolved to find out for himself.

The Origins of the Method

All he had to go on was that his friends had noticed that, during a performance, his breathing was audible – he sucked in air through his mouth. Normal speaking did not seem to affect his voice. He therefore placed himself in front of a mirror to see if he could distinguish between his manner of 'doing' in the two situations. When he started to recite he noticed that he tended to pull his head back, depress his throat and suck in air through his mouth in such a way as to produce a gasping sound. Later, when he was able to observe his normal speaking more closely he saw that these three tendencies were still present but to a less marked degree; when the demands of recitation were great they were exaggerated further. This served to confirm his conjecture that it was what he *did* when reciting which lay at the root of the problem. Furthermore, after a few months of experimentation the one thing he found he could, to some degree, reduce directly – the pulling back of his head – had an indirect effect on the pressure on his throat and the gasping; and his tendency to hoarseness decreased (on examination his doctor noted much less inflammation of his larynx and vocal cords).

FOCUSING ON THE PRIMARY CONTROL

Having confirmed a clear link between the way he held his head and the effect on his voice – between what he termed *use* and *functioning* – Alexander continued his experiments. He found that if he moved his head forward a *little* his voice improved further. He also discovered that if he went too far, he put his head forward and *down*, and this was just as harmful to his vocal mechanism as his habitual tendency to pull it *back* and *down*: either extreme exerted undue pressure on his larynx. At the same time he began to notice that there was a whole pattern of *misuse* that was not confined to his neck and head but included his tendency to raise his chest and hollow and 'narrow' his lower back (thereby shortening his stature). The resulting muscular tension spread all the way down to his legs and toes (he recalled with some sense of irony a former drama teacher's advice to 'take hold of the floor with his feet'!). Somehow he had to find a way of maintaining a lengthening stature that would require his head to go forward and *up*, his spine to lengthen – without lifting his chest – and his back to widen.

IDENTIFYING FAULTY KINAESTHESIA

When Alexander tried to maintain this new lengthened stature while reciting he was surprised to discover that it appeared to be impossible. Enlisting the help of two extra mirrors to monitor his movements, he found that at the critical moment (when he came to recite) he was still pulling his head back and down, as before. He realized that he had been working from the assumption that he only had to *will* a certain thing and it would automatically happen. Was his failure peculiar to him? As he observed others it became more and more apparent to him that it is practically a universal delusion to believe that we can change habitual ways of doing merely by wishing to do them differently.

Finally it dawned on Alexander that he had been depending upon the way his body felt – a disconcertingly unreliable gauge. Discouraged as he was, he began at this point (1894) to get an inkling that he was onto something really important: *'I got the idea of what it really was and could be. If it is possible for feeling to become untrustworthy as a means of direction, it should also be possible to make it trustworthy again.'*

One of Alexander's passions was for reciting Shakespeare and he had often found inspiration in the characterization of human potential expressed in *Hamlet* (II. ii. 316):

What a piece of work is a man, how noble in reason, how
infinite in faculties, in form and moving how express and
admirable, in action how like an angel, in apprehension
how like a god: the beauty of the world, the paragon of
animals . . .

In discussing with his father what he was now aware of in himself
and others he began pondering the fact that there is no
difference between us and the dog or cat in that we do not *know*
how to use ourselves well. Puzzling over his observations in an
evolutionary framework, he began to wonder whether it might
not be the case that man's capacity to live with himself was out
of step with his ability to manipulate his environment. In
particular, reliance on 'instinctive' control seemed more and
more unsatisfactory. What was needed, he believed, was a more
conscious and rational approach to restoring co-ordination.

THINKING IN ACTIVITY
The problems – force of habit and faulty kinaesthesia – were
triggered whenever Alexander decided to use his voice. In
Pavlovian terms, the *stimulus* of recitation always invoked the
same, habitual *response*. He argued to himself that if it were
possible to prevent his unsatisfactory reaction to the *idea* of
reciting – by deciding not to act on his intention to recite
(inhibition and non-doing) – then it must be possible to find the
new direction necessary to maintain the proper relationship
between neck, head and back while reciting (or during any other
activity). He therefore practised *consciously* projecting directions
from his brain to the relevant parts of his body. In this way, he
reasoned that the co-ordination necessary to avoid the
interference with his breathing and vocal mechanism might be
secured.

He found, however, that at the critical moment when he came
to speak or recite he would stop giving directions and revert to
his old pattern, which continued to 'feel' right to him even
though he could *see* that it was wrong. After many unsatisfactory
attempts he decided that for a while he would merely practise

giving himself the directions without trying to 'do' them or follow on with speaking. He wrote:

> I would give the new directions in front of the mirror for long periods together, for successive days and weeks and sometimes even months, without attempting to do them, and the experience I gained in giving these directions proved of great value when the time came for me to consider how to put them into practice.

What Alexander had been working on was an example of what the American philosopher and educator John Dewey called 'thinking in activity': being able to link more and more directions together in the proper sequence ('one after the other and all together') so that they can inform a particular activity.

Alexander made further unsuccessful attempts to maintain this 'directed' use of himself while reciting. Analysing what had gone wrong he came to the conclusion that he had been attempting a new use of his body, which was bound to feel wrong, and at the same time trusting to what felt right to indicate whether he was employing his new use correctly. His mirrors told him how unreliable his body sense was.

AN END TO END-GAINING
The procedure that finally worked was this. Instead of following his intention to speak or recite with the action of speaking or reciting – which always invoked the habitual pattern of misuse – at the critical moment he would stop and reconsider his decision, *all the while continuing to project the directions for his new, improved use.* He would stop and say to himself, 'Shall I:

- not go on to speak that sentence – in other words, do nothing; or
- do something entirely different, for example, raise my arm; or
- go on to speak the sentence while giving the directions?'

By choosing to do nothing or to go for a different end in the *majority* of cases he was eventually able to maintain with consistency the proper use of himself while reciting. Confirmation that, at last, he was on the right track came when he became entirely free of his throat and vocal troubles. The various respiratory and nasal problems he had suffered, from since childhood also cleared up.

Alexander's Teaching Career

Alexander resumed his acting career for a while but very soon became totally involved in teaching. First he taught other actors about the 'use of the self' on which good vocal technique is founded; then, increasingly, he worked with chronic cases referred by doctors. His reputation grew quickly. His brother, Alfred, also joined him in the work. A prominent surgeon in Sydney, convinced that the Technique had universal value, encouraged Alexander to go to London where the Technique might reach a wider public.

He arrived in London in 1904 armed with letters of introduction to doctors and others, but it was within the theatrical profession that he made his name as a teacher in those early years in London: most of the leading actors of the day consulted him. While Alexander's work was always held in high regard by certain doctors, it was the general public to whom he appealed. He wrote letters to the press on the shortcomings of the deep breathing exercises then in vogue, pamphlets describing his Technique and, in 1910, published his first book, *Man's Supreme Inheritance*; it stayed in print throughout his lifetime (and has been republished in recent years). By 1914 FM, who had always used his hands to try to convey what verbal instruction along could not, was developing a more sensitive use of his hands, making possible an entirely different kind of change than ordinary postural adjustment. With the onset of the First World War, opportunities for refining his manual skills were limited. He began visiting the USA on a regular basis and soon built up a large practice there, assisted by his brother. This American connection proved important for many reasons, not least of which was his meeting with John Dewey.

THE DEWEY CONNECTION

Dewey began having lessons in the Technique in 1916 and he continued to do so at intervals throughout his life. Dewey wrote the Forewords to three of Alexander's books and proofread *Constructive Conscious Control of the Individual* (1923). He found in Alexander's work practical confirmation of some of the philosophical concepts he had been wrestling with: the unity of mind and body and the role of inhibition in behaviour, for instance. Dewey's writings are so permeated with his knowledge and experience of the Alexander Technique that it could be argued that a prerequisite of understanding Dewey would be to have lessons in the Technique!

Dewey was also instrumental in giving Frank Pierce Jones the encouragement to undertake basic research into the mechanism of the Technique (see Chapter 4). And, remarkably, Dewey expressed the opinion that 'the Alexander Technique bears the same relationship to education . . . that education bears to all other activities.'

CRITIQUE OF STANDARD EDUCATIONAL METHODS

Alexander often referred to the need for a different kind of education. The question was, and is: How might children be helped to learn more effectively? Can they be freed from excessive tensions and come through schooling with their intrinsic co-ordination relatively unimpaired? In 1924 a little school was set up outside London 'upon the principle', Alexander wrote, 'that the end for which they are working is of minor importance as compared with the way they direct the use of themselves for the gaining of that end'. The pupils were of primary school age with learning difficulties, and were the children of parents having Alexander lessons. The curriculum was of the usual kind and the day-to-day running of the school was in the charge of Alexander's assistants. The school had to close in 1942, all the pupils having been evacuated to the USA early in the Second World War. To my knowledge no detailed account exists of its achievements and shortcomings, but it seems to have worked well. Since then there have been occasional incursions of Alexander's ideas into schools, but nothing of any lasting success. One of the difficulties lay in grafting what are actually quite radical and challenging ideas – not least for the teachers concerned – onto institutions which tend to be, for the most part, resistant to change.

Fruition

The 1930s saw the summit of achievement of the Technique in Alexander's lifetime. Alexander's third book, *The Use of the Self*, was published in 1932. It proved to be the most popular of his books in the UK. Many famous people took lessons, including Aldous Huxley and George Bernard Shaw, both of whom were enthusiastic advocates. Alexander also began to train teachers in the Technique. Around this time (according to Lulie Westfeldt, one of the first teachers Alexander trained), his skill in making changes in people through his hands took a quantum leap. Frank Pierce Jones, commenting on this, reports how Alexander claimed he was able to get the same results in three daily lessons as had taken him three weeks previously. Almost immediately Alexander could produce that unique experience of freedom, ease and lightness of movement – the hallmark of the Technique – without having to concern himself very much with how much the pupil understood of the theory behind it. This could and can be a mixed blessing, as we shall see in Chapter 5: it carries the danger that the Technique becomes yet another form of treatment – the pupil taking little responsibility for creating and maintaining change within himself.

DEFENDING THE CAUSE

The story of the development of the Technique would be incomplete without some mention of the libel action which Alexander brought in South Africa in 1945. Frank Pierce Jones summarizes the main points succinctly and entertainingly: the case had its farcical side and it illuminated aspects of Alexander's character and the often unholy alliance between the state and the medical establishment.

Ernst Jokl – a physician, expert in exercise physiology and

physical education officer of the South African government, published in collaboration with a colleague an attack on Alexander and his followers. The editorial, which appeared in an official journal of the South African government, was entitled 'Quackery versus Physical Education'. Alexander was caricatured as an 'Australian gym master' and compared unfavourably to Mary Baker Eddy (the founder of Christian Science) and African witch doctors; the assertion was made that the 'legendary "primary control" . . . enables man to subject the work of his internal organs to the supervision of his will'. Alexander had never made claims of that sort: on the contrary, the aim of his Technique was to ensure that those aspects of functioning that are mainly involuntary, such as digestion and breathing, should *not* be interfered with; nor had he claimed to cure cancer or appendicitis, as Jokl maintained.

It seems that what precipitated the attacks was the possibility that the Alexander Technique might supplant the physical education given to South African school children. The president of the Transvaal Teachers' Association had advocated the Alexander Technique, warning that physical training, deep breathing and relaxation exercises were probably harmful. This had incensed Jokl and his colleague, who thought this 'a most shocking proposal' and 'a very serious threat to the health of school children'. The case finally came to court in 1948. Alexander won large damages and was satisfied that his reputation and that of his work had been substantiated. The libel action was not, however, without its costs. Alexander's legal expenses were barely covered by the award and the process leading up to the trial had taxed his health severely. In 1947, aged 77, he had a bad fall and a week later a stroke, paralysing his left hand and leg and the left side of his face. He won his case, but it might have been better for him to have ignored the attack.

Within a few months he had recovered from the effects of the stroke and was working harder than ever before. He continued to give private lessons and to supervise the teacher training course until 1955 when, after a chill incurred at a race meeting (he regularly bet on horses) he took to his bed and died a week later, aged 86.

Alexander's Legacy

Alexander did not name a successor to carry on his teaching. An umbrella organization the Society of Teachers of the Alexander Technique (STAT) came into being to oversee teacher training courses – run by some of the teachers Alexander had trained – to maintain a register of teachers who had undergone an approved training course and to provide information for the general public. In 1965 there were just 37 teachers – members of the Society – practising worldwide. By 1992 this had swollen to over 500 teachers in the UK alone and a similar number abroad. Still more teachers are registered with national societies affiliated to STAT. The Technique is increasingly popular – articles on it appear frequently in the press – and more and more people know of it and are taking lessons.

Long before there was much interest in alternatives to orthodox medicine, Alexander was promulgating and teaching his ideas on the essential unity of mind and body; how a clear and rational understanding of the link between the two could be of great benefit to the whole person. The Technique still stands on its own merits amid the plethora of mind/body and healing methods that have flourished in recent years.

Chapter 4

How the Technique Works

This story of perceptiveness, of intelligence, and of persistence, shown by a man without medical training, is one of the true epics of medical research and practice.

N. Tinbergen, Nobel Laureate in Physiology and Medicine, 1973

Mr Alexander has done a service to the subject [will and reflex action] by insistently treating each act as involving the whole integrated individual, the whole psycho-physical man. To take a step is an affair, not of this or that limb solely, but of the total neuro-muscular activity of the moment – not least of the head and neck.

Sir Charles Sherrington, physiologist, 1946

After studying over a period of years Mr Alexander's method in actual operation, I would stake myself upon the fact that he has applied to our ideas and beliefs about ourselves and about our acts, exactly the same method of experimentation and of production of new sensory observations, as tests and means of developing thought, that have been the source of all progress in the physical sciences . . .

John Dewey, philosopher and educationalist, 1924

The men who made these statements staked their reputations on the validity of the Alexander Technique. Impressive though these testimonials are, however, they do not represent evidence that the Alexander Technique works.

To some, the principles of the Technique are self-evident. This was Alexander's position: he carried out the work on himself in the first place and then found corroboration for his discoveries over the course of 60 years of teaching others. The basic propositions can be demonstrated readily in the teaching situation, according to Raymond Dart, Professor of Anatomy at the University of Witwatersrand, South Africa (one of the few scientists who has taken the trouble to investigate the Technique scientifically). This implies, of course, that the Technique cannot simply be taken 'off the shelf' by anyone but is crucially dependent on the skilled intervention of a teacher.

There are three areas of research that have been carried out with regard to the Technique: evidence for the 'operational ideas' – the primary control, inhibition and direction; evidence that improvement in use can affect functioning; and work on the efficacy of different methods of teaching the Technique.

Evidence for the Operational Ideas

THE PRIMARY CONTROL

Disturbance of the primary control can be observed and measured in the laboratory by eliciting the *startle reflex* (see Figure 5). Alexander teacher Frank Pierce Jones has shown, using experimental psychology methods, that the response to an unexpectedly loud noise is an increase in muscle tension – first in the large neck muscles, then, over half a second, spreading through the trunk to the legs.[1] As for posture, the neck stiffens and pokes forward, the head retracts and the chin thrusts forward, the shoulders raise, the arms extend, the chest depresses and the legs flex. Jones also noted that when the sound was just loud enough to elicit a response, it would appear only in the neck muscles and nowhere else. He conjectured that the stooping seen in old age might be, in large part, the cumulative effect of many years' unrelieved responses to stressful situations.

'The evidence that the neck plays a critical role in posture is overwhelming'[2] according to physiologist Professor Abrahams. It was previously thought that the main control for posture and

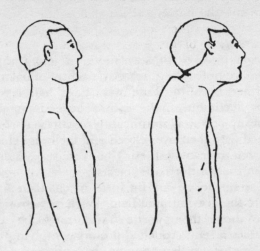

Figure 5: The startle reflex: The common reaction to stress starts
with a tightening of the neck muscles. The increase of tension
then spreads throughout the body

balance lay in inputs from the semi-circular canals of the inner
ear. We now know that the sub-occipital muscles – the small
deep muscles of the neck, important for maintaining the poise
of the head on the neck – have a higher density of nerve
receptors ('muscle spindles' – which give information to the
brain about the condition of those muscles) than any other
muscle in the body. If a local anaesthetic is injected into the sub-
occipital muscles on one side of the neck – putting them out
of action – the subject struggles to maintain his balance,
tending to list over to that side and walking like a drunken
person.

The 'righting reaction' in cats also provides supporting
evidence for the existence of the primary control: if a cat is
dropped upside down from a height, the combined inputs from
the neck and inner ear quickly bring the cat into an upright
position so that it lands safely on its feet – the head leading, the

body following (though I would not recommend you try this experiment on the family cat!).

The Anti-gravity Response

How do we manage to stay more or less upright? Many observers have noted that the body's centre of balance tends to move further back in those who have had lessons in the Alexander Technique. *Sway analyses* have demonstrated that Alexander subjects sway significantly less than 'normal' subjects when tested with their eyes closed and their legs close together, implying that their kinaesthetic ('body sense') system functions better than that of normal subjects.[3]

There seems to be an intrinsic mechanism operating in response to the gravitational field. Work on astronauts in zero gravity has shown the opposite of what might be expected: the body assumes a semi-crouched position, implying that gravity naturally produces a 'lengthening' or 'anti-gravity' response.[4] As yet, not enough is known about the various bio-mechanical elements that contribute to upright posture. Certainly the spinal curves, properly maintained, have an important part to play, aided by the properties of the intervertebral discs, the ligaments and other soft tissue support of the spine as well as the active lengthening of muscle. All this appears to give a certain springy, elastic quality to the spine which can be felt through an Alexander teacher's hands and which is experienced by a subject as an energizing 'upflow', producing lighter and easier movement.

INHIBITION AND DIRECTION

When an impulse to act in some way arises and a decision is made to act on that impulse, programs are activated from the back part of the brain – the cerebellum. The cerebellum contains a huge repertoire of all previously-undertaken movement patterns. Impulses are constantly arising spontaneously of which we are not (initially) conscious. Ben Libet, Professor of Physiology at the University of California, has carried out work that appears to throw light on the brain mechanisms corresponding to Alexander's 'critical moment' – the point at which he could prevent himself from getting 'set' to recite. What Libet found is that we have just over one tenth of a second when the window of our consciousness registers the impulse. In that time there is the opportunity to veto the reaction which would otherwise automatically follow.[5,6] That does not sound very much time – and indeed it is not – but an alert subject can readily be trained so as not to miss the moment.

Recent work by Alexander teacher and physiologist Stevens and colleagues has shown how the Alexander-guided movement from sitting to standing is a more efficient movement than is normally the case.[7] Subjects habitually stiffen their necks, pull their heads back and down and increase the tension of trunk flexion and extension muscles: that is, they pull themselves badly downwards in the effort to go upwards. Using a force gauge platform, measurements of muscle activity and special movement photographs, Alexander-guided movement was shown to involve less downward pressure, less muscular effort and a quicker, more vertical movement. Subjects report a greater sense of ease because there is less interference with breathing and the movement is lighter. The relative effortlessness of a directed movement is associated with a more appropriate lengthening use of the trunk musculature.

For most of this century, the consensus among neurophysiologists was that we can only 'think' of movement in a rather non-specific way. Yet this separation between 'thinking' and 'doing' has been challenged by work that has shown that subjects can not only control individual muscles but can also narrow down their control to a single nerve supplying a number of microscopic muscle fibres![8]

The efficacy of the Alexander Technique in identifying links between attention, intention and body use therefore has support from a range of scientific studies.

Evidence that Use Affects Functioning

MUSCLE FIBRE TYPES

In human beings there is roughly a 50/50 balance between the millions of red and white muscle fibres that make up muscle (compare the red meat of beef and the white meat of poultry). The red muscle fibres, active in slow, rhythmical movement and in maintaining posture, tend not to fatigue. White muscle fibres are recruited in quick, powerful movement and tire quickly when used. There is evidence of a greater preponderance of red fibres in the deeper muscle layers, which are believed to be more concerned with postural support, than in the superficial layers involved with expression and movement.

Sitting for any length of time produces a vicious cycle of slumping and over-contraction in most people. The office worker who regularly 'works out' – without a basic program of gentle, slow, rhythmical movement – is likely to produce a deterioration in body use and functioning – quite the opposite, of course, of what is intended. What is probably happening is that, once white fibres tend to be overemployed (as they will be in those people who regularly take vigorous exercise), fatigue will set in and more white muscle fibres will be recruited to try to avoid further collapse.

KINAESTHESIA

David Garlick, Senior Lecturer in Physiology at the University of New South Wales, Australia, uses the expression 'the lost sixth sense' to describe how our kinaesthetic sense seems to have become lost or suppressed in modern civilization (Alexander described this as 'faulty sensory appreciation').[9] Garlick relates this to the finite capacity of the brain – in an over-stimulating world – to process the large amounts of information that come from all sources: the outside world, our internal thoughts and feelings, and the excessive amount of muscular activity that seems to be involved in 'doing'. Too much of this information can block out the potentially rich inputs from our sixth sense about the tone of our muscles, subtle shifts in body orientation and in the relationships between different parts of the body.

During fast movement there less opportunity for the inputs from the sixth sense to be registered consciously which might allow modification of the movement pattern. On the other hand, slow movements, such as those that occur in T'ai Chi and Feldenkrais (see Chapter 6) allow time for feedback – and therefore for the quality of movement to be improved. Once a movement pattern can be executed perfectly, then it can be speeded up without loss of co-ordination.

BREATHING AND STATES OF MIND

Research has shown that Alexander-trained subjects breathe on average 10 times per minute and more deeply than untrained subjects who average 18 times per minute, more shallowly. [10] In Alexander subjects there is more active muscle tone in the extensor muscles of the back and reduced tone in the flexor muscles of the front of the torso. In untrained subjects, when the back muscles are not working properly there is excessive tension in the abdominal and chest muscles. This excessive tension interferes with breathing.

Differences in breathing patterns of this order have implications for a person's mood and ability to maintain calm in stressful circumstances (the panic reactions associated with hyperventilation are more likely to be prevented with Alexander training). There is good evidence that mood states are accompanied by changes in muscle tone. The person who is depressed emotionally is usually physically depressed as well: slumping is associated with loss of tone in the extensor muscles, and the head, neck and torso droop forward. In anger, chest and abdominal muscles are over-contracted. Anxiety is held in over-tense muscles all over the body but is localized particularly in the neck, shoulders and forehead. In all these mood states, breathing is impaired. After a while a person may become quite unaware of the state of his muscles. Circumstances may change but the emotional state may persist.

An important function of Alexander lessons is sometimes to help increase awareness of how emotional states can be frozen in certain physical attitudes; it may then be easier to let go of inappropriate feelings and begin the process of change.

BLOOD-PRESSURE

One small study found evidence to suggest that members of a symphony orchestra, suffering from stress and raised blood-pressure and given a basic course of Alexander lessons, showed a similar drop in blood-pressure as other orchestra members receiving drug treatment, compared with other groups who received nothing (the 'control' group) or who ran 4½ miles (7 km) three times a week. [11] The crucial distinction between those who received Alexander lessons and those who were treated with drugs, however, was that the latter felt that their performance seemed to be impaired by the drugs, whereas the 'Alexandered' musicians reported more satisfaction with their performance.

There is a further consideration in relation to blood-pressure. The stressed individual who feels driven to take vigorous exercise in an attempt to feel better and more relaxed will probably add to his already high level of muscle tension and make more effort than is necessary for the exercise being undertaken. A young person will probably not notice any immediate consequences, but the question arises whether – even in a young person – it makes sense to stress the heart unduly (definitely inadvisable in an older person).

POSTURAL CHANGES

The specialist in physical medicine and Alexander teacher W. Barlow carried out a study on army recruits to measure how much they pulled back their heads as they moved to sit down. [12] He found that the majority pulled their heads back by at least an inch. Very few could tell that they were doing so even when they were asked to give particular attention to this shortening. On being asked to prevent the shortening, most still retracted the head even though they believed that they were not. This provides some confirmation of Alexander's observations of the unreliability of body sense.

Dr Barlow also surveyed students of speech and drama. His

study found that over 80 per cent had substantial or severe postural defects. Ongoing study showed either no improvement or actual deterioration of the students' posture during their course, following the specific remedial exercises prescribed. The control group – students at a music college who received Alexander lessons – demonstrated significant improvement in their posture during their training. More importantly, the student musicians' level of performance was higher than would otherwise have been expected.

CASE HISTORIES

Alexander and Barlow cite an impressive number and wide variety of cases where the Technique appears to have worked – or to have been the decisive factor in improvement. The trouble is that any amount of anecdotal evidence – individual case histories – is not in itself conclusive: other variables could be at work. These case histories, however, do point to the need for further research.

Research into Ways of Teaching the Technique

There is clearly a need to evaluate the effectiveness of different teaching methods.

Informal 'research' is being carried out all the time in every Alexander lesson (each one being an experimental situation). This began with Alexander's early discovery that words alone were not enough to produce proper change. There are a number of components that need to mesh successfully for learning in the fullest sense to take place. The teacher constantly observes the effects of his hands on the pupil to see whether the release that should be occurring is actually taking place. A good teacher will draw on a repertoire of ways of communicating about the Technique: as well as touch, he will use demonstration and call on images, ideas and language that can make sense to pupils from a wide range of backgrounds, life experiences and interests. The outcome is that there is now a great diversity of ways of teaching the Technique. Some of these are discussed in the next chapter.

Chapter 5

Learning the Technique

There are three ways to learn the Alexander Technique: reading about it, participating in a group workshop, and/or taking private lessons.

Reading About It

Reading about the Technique and studying the ideas can be helpful. For me, it opened up a new world and inspired me to want to go deeply into the Technique and to undertake a teacher training course (see the Further Reading section of this book).

Louise Morgan, the first person other than Alexander himself to write a book on the Technique (*Inside Yourself* – long out of print) claimed to have applied it successfully by studying Alexander's books. Alexander declared that if anyone was prepared to do what he did – described in detail in *The Use of the Self* – he or she could manage without a teacher. It could be argued that anyone who had really gained something would have no need to consult a teacher; and there is no way of conclusively proving a negative. Alexander teachers, however, have good reason to be sceptical about the likelihood of anyone – independent of a teacher's guidance – being able to make any substantial and worthwhile change by himself. People who have tried on their own soon realize that they are not getting very far. It is not easy, even with the help of a competent teacher, to change the habits of a lifetime. To enter wholly unknown realms of experience – letting go of the familiar – is something very few of us manage unaided.

Workshops

An increasing number of group workshops are now offered introducing the ideas of the Technique with a little practical work. They can be a relatively inexpensive and non-committal way of finding out about the Technique: you will also be hearing about it 'from the horse's mouth'. Many people enjoy the social aspect of a group and it can be instructive to be shown shared patterns of misuse – as well as what may be done to alter them. Usually there are opportunities for *some* individual experience of the Technique, especially if you are prepared to act as a guinea-pig. Attending a workshop can help you to decide whether you want to take private lessons from a particular teacher or perhaps to investigate the Technique further with another teacher.

The down side of group work is that the amount of individual, hands-on experience is going to be limited by the size of the group, the time available and the need for the teacher(s) to maintain group involvement. Changes in body use can be demonstrated in the workshop, but the 'thinking in activity' which is necessary to enable someone to become fully independent of a teacher cannot be properly learned in this context. This is because there will not be enough opportunity at an introductory level to link the experience of being directed by the teacher's hands to your own process of inhibition and direction-giving.

The main value of a group, therefore, is to introduce you to the Technique. More than the equivalent of two day-long workshops, unless there is a low student/teacher ratio, is stretching it unless you want a lot of chat and 'skirmishing in the foothills'. An exception might be a week's holiday course: the 'retreat' formula on a Greek island often appeals, although it may be worth enquiring how many individual lessons or their equivalents you can expect. And, given the cost of such a holiday, wouldn't you rather invest in a sizable basic course of individual lessons?

One group format which can go beyond the superficial is the specialist workshop, for example those given for musicians or other performing artists. Here problems of preparation and performance can be usefully explored in the light thrown on them by the Alexander Technique.

Finally, some teachers hold regular small group meetings for their private pupils. This can be a welcome chance to share experiences with other people who may be at different stages of learning the Technique.

Individual Lessons

Private lessons are indispensable if you want to discover the lasting value of the Technique in improving the quality of many aspects of your life. In lessons, the teacher's hands subtly guide the way your body is organized so that movement becomes lighter, freer and easier. You become much more aware of tensions you may have been creating, how to let go of them and how to maintain improvement.

The range of problems and situations that might be helped by lessons have already been mentioned in Chapter 1; mostly, this comprises the numerous health problems that can be brought on by body misuse. A growing category of people who are drawn to the Technique includes those who are interested in personal development; they are likely to be concerned with the *preventive* aspects of the Technique and with enjoying life with less of the normal decline in vigour and capacity as they grow older.

MAKING A COMMITMENT

Before starting lessons you might ask yourself what level of commitment to the Technique you want to make. This can be discussed on the phone, but an introductory lesson may be necessary so that you can find out more. A minimum number of sessions may be recommended in order for you to give the Technique a fair trial.

However many lessons you finally take, you should be clear from the outset that *the lasting benefits of the Technique come from making it your own.* The teacher – however skilled in the use of his hands – cannot do it all for you. You won't be 'put right' and then not have to think about it in your daily life! The Technique is not a course of treatment to which you submit yourself passively. It requires a willingness to take responsibility for your own condition, whatever its causes. In the course of lessons you will begin to discover what you are doing to yourself to cause pain or to limit your mobility or capacity to learn and function well. Your teacher will suggest that you find time most days of the week for a short rest and a little work on yourself; and that you aim to become more and more conscious of *how* you approach your daily tasks.

The biggest commitment, then, is not just the financial but the personal one: do you really want to change? As has often been observed, most people say they want to change and yet remain the same.

WHOSE PROBLEM IS IT, ANYWAY?
Psychoanalysts have drawn our attention to the phenomenon of 'secondary gain': that is, that a patient's symptoms – however painful – may resist treatment because they bring certain benefits to the patient. For example, someone suffering from arthritis may live with someone in a mutually advantageous being cared for/taking care of relationship, a status quo that would be disturbed were the arthritic person to recover. All Alexander teachers have worked with people who seem to 'need' their symptoms. Sometimes it appears that lessons are used to confirm the 'hopelessness' of their condition. This frequently occurs if someone's partner has the idea that it would be good for him to take a course of lessons; usually the person comes under duress and is not motivated to change.

Children come into a special category. We do not know how much of the Technique can be learned consciously by children. The most important influences on them are probably the models they see before them: principally their parents and teachers. Children are often brought by parents anxious that their child may be acquiring their own problems, postural or otherwise; there is also always the danger that lessons may be seen by the child as yet another indication of where he does not measure up to his parent's expectations. It may be suggested, therefore, that the parents think first of taking lessons for themselves.

If the child is young it is better to start in a low-key way, with the child sharing a small part of the parents' lessons. A seed may be sown; later on the child may want more time in the lessons for himself. Problems start at an early age and children who have had some gentle and positive exposure to the Technique in their formative years will be at an advantage. At the same time, a child's development is to a large degree about forming a sense of self: the Technique may challenge aspects of this and may not, therefore, always be welcomed. However, a frequent refrain from pupils starting lessons in the second half of their lives is: *if only* I had come across the Technique when I was at school – I am sure my life would have been quite different.

CHOOSING A TEACHER
You will probably start by personal recommendation – but even then what may suit one may not suit another. Make sure, at least, that the teacher has undergone an approved three-year training course. In the UK, the Society of Teachers of the Alexander Technique (STAT) maintains a register of teaching members; abroad, many other countries have their own national teachers' societies affiliated to STAT (see the Useful Addresses section of this book).

If there are a number of teachers in your locality, it may be wise to take a lesson or two from more than one teacher before you commit yourself to a course of lessons. Factors you may want to consider, apart from fees, are the teacher's experience, personality and gender and the content and style of teaching.

Trust and *confidence* are important in any professional relationship. The Technique involves touch, mostly on the head and neck and limbs but also on the torso. Although you will not need to remove your clothes (your teacher will be able to feel and observe patterns of use through your clothing), many people may naturally feel somewhat vulnerable in their first few lessons. A woman may feel safer with another woman. You may feel an instant rapport with a teacher, or you may feel he is on a different wavelength. If you don't get on so well with a particular teacher, premature conclusions about the value of the Technique may be misplaced. (Later on you may find that liking your teacher has little relation to how much you can learn from him!)

Many teachers will have pursued another profession or occupation prior to becoming an Alexander teacher, or they may have developed expertise in special areas. Strictly speaking this should not matter greatly, because the most important thing is the basic core of Alexander teaching. Nevertheless, if a teacher is, for instance, a musician, he will clearly have a dimension of knowledge, experience and empathy to bring to bear on a particular pupil's difficulties in that area. The violin, viola and flute are examples of very demanding instruments: a teacher's clear understanding of the technical problems and any compromises that may have to be made may prove indispensable.

LESSON DETAILS
Now, what about the practical details? Cost, length, frequency, number and so on?

Cost
The price of lessons varies enormously. A recently qualified teacher may charge less and give more time. In the UK fees vary between approximately £12 and £25 at the time of writing (1992), for a lesson lasting between 30 and 45 minutes. This seems to be about the right length of time for an adequate amount of experience and information to be imparted without overloading the pupil. Some teachers offer concessionary fees to students or people on low incomes; it is always worth enquiring about any possible discounts.

When you make appointments for lessons, it should be made clear whether a cancellation fee will be charged if adequate notice is not given. If emergencies keep cropping up or you find yourself arriving consistently late for appointments you may need to ask yourself whether it really is the right time to be taking lessons. This can save both you and your teacher unnecessary aggravation and means that it will be easier to resume lessons at a later date in a positive atmosphere.

Frequency and Number

All teachers will suggest a higher frequency of regular lessons initially. Progress will be slow and faltering if there are wide gaps between lessons in the early stages: the beneficial effects of lessons are less likely to be consolidated under the normal stresses of daily life and the habits of a lifetime! Alexander advised *daily* lessons for a few weeks as a basic course of instruction. His fee was quite high – the equivalent of a private medical consultation; possibly he thought that people wouldn't take his work seriously unless it was seen to be as valuable as orthodox medicine. Alternatively, perhaps, he put a high price on the skills he had laboured so long and hard to acquire. There are now many more teachers who are interested in reaching a wider population base and whose fees are much lower. Also it is not so practicable for most people to come daily nor, perhaps, is it so desirable: time is needed to assimilate and consolidate the changes made in lessons.

A reasonable compromise might be having lessons twice a week for a month, then weekly for a couple of months, then less often still. An occasional reminder or a 'top-up' course of a handful of lessons from time to time may be desirable. Some people, however, will need to come three times a week at first. For others in less dire straits once a week may be adequate.

Most people will need approximately 20 lessons or more to make substantial improvement in their condition and to establish a sound base from which to maintain progress. This may sound rather daunting and expensive; don't let it put you off. It is no more costly than a week's holiday. Think how much you spend on your car – and yet the benefits of a course of Alexander lessons can last the rest of your life.

If you don't think you can afford to come frequently enough at first it may be better to wait until you feel you can, rather than starting in an unsatisfactory way.

A QUICK FIX OR LIFE SENTENCE?

In the final analysis you should consider carefully what you want from Alexander lessons. This is something you might want to discuss with your teacher at the first session, if not before. Your rate of change cannot be forced: to make progress you need time, repeated experience of improved body use and a fair amount of intelligent effort on your part. A useful analogy is to think of your body as a musical instrument: it needs to be tuned regularly and played often (if only for short periods of time) for satisfactory performance. (How many musicians wanting to achieve optimum performance would abuse their instruments in the way we abuse our bodies?)

Many people are only interested in a modest level of competence and improved functioning. An example is the taxi driver who came for lessons complaining of disabling headaches. It quickly became apparent that their major cause was the way he jammed his head back and down, especially when driving. After three lessons he was clear enough about the problem to be able to inhibit a *small part* of his tendency to tighten his neck and retract his head; his use, though poor, was improved sufficiently to reduce his headaches and to permit him to drive unimpaired for long enough to carry on his work. At the other extreme are Alexander teachers: they will often continue refining their skills, with the help of more senior teachers, even though they have already had the equivalent of many hundreds of hours of private lessons. It is up to you how far you want to take the Technique.

WHAT TO EXPECT

When you come for your first lesson your teacher will ask you a few details about yourself, such as your occupation, age, any relevant medical history and whether you have sought help elsewhere. People often don't realize quite what the Technique involves. They may have heard it might help with back pain, for example, and may expect all the work to be done *for* them. Alternatively the Technique may be the last port of call for those who have done the rounds of other practitioners and have finally come to the conclusion that it may be within *their* power to effect improvement in their condition.

Alexander teachers are not trained in medical diagnosis and will therefore suggest, as appropriate, that you seek a medical opinion of some kind if you have not already done so. They will neither offer a cure nor commit themselves to a prognosis. The task is one of re-education. Each person, whatever his presenting problems, will follow *in broad outline* a similar path of instruction.

You won't need to undress but you should wear unrestrictive clothing – a tight skirt or jeans will obviously make it hard to bend your legs freely or comfortably.

THE FIRST LESSON

What happens in the first lesson? *This varies in detail from teacher to teacher, so what follows is a rough guide.* As well as clarifying your expectations for the Technique, your teacher will probably explain a little of the Technique's background and the importance of the primary control to co-ordination generally. The teacher may illustrate this point by having you get into or out of a chair (when the stiffening of the neck and head retraction are nearly always exaggerated), or he may take a brief look at a particular activity you have problems with.

A substantial part of the first lesson may well involve what may be called 'lying down, releasing work'. This involves resting on your back on a couch with your head supported by a couple of paperback books or so, legs bent, feet resting flat and knees pointing up to the ceiling. This makes it easier at first to allow the necessary release and lengthening of the body. The teacher will do this for you in the lesson by touch and by moving and repositioning parts of your body gently and slowly. He will also show you how to begin working on yourself.

The idea of inhibition/non-doing will be introduced. For example, the teacher may say, 'I am just going to raise your leg and I would like you to let me take it for you.' Most pupils, at first, will be unable to resist the temptation to lift the leg or will even increase the level of tension in order *not* to lift it! Gradually

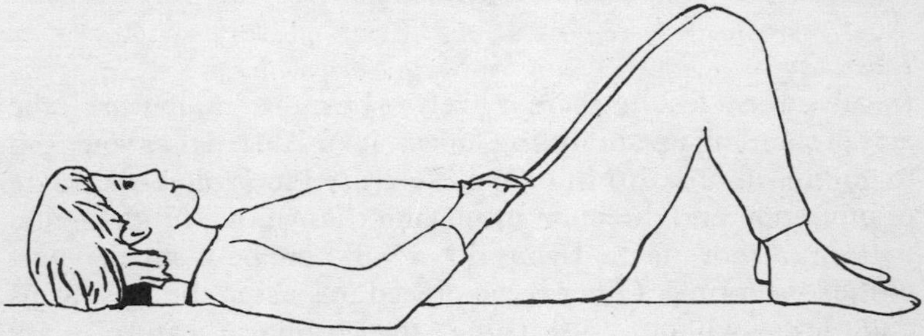

Figure 6: The lying down, releasing position

you learn to avoid doing more than is needed.

The process of giving directions comes next. You will discover – with the help of the teacher's hands initially – that merely to *think* of allowing your leg to release out of your hip, for example, will allow it to move easily and freely. This is the crucial difference between *trying* to do something and *allowing* it to happen. The teacher will return constantly to the primary control prior to and during the adjustment of another part of your body, gently encouraging the release of your head from your neck so that your spine lengthens and back widens and flattens out on the couch.

Your 'homework' will be to set aside 10 to 20 minutes – in the middle of the day if possible, otherwise when you get in from work – to lie down on a firm but comfortable surface (a thickly-carpeted floor is ideal) to help 'undo' some of the tensions that have developed during the day. Don't expect such a marked experience of release on your own as you will probably have had in your lesson. Regardless of whether you are able to give these directions very effectively at first, you will experience many benefits. Some people notice some relief, for instance from back pain, immediately; others find after two or three weeks that if they miss lying down for two or three days it makes a noticeable difference to their ease and comfort.

Later Stages

In subsequent lessons there is likely to be more 'chair-work': the acts of standing up and sitting 'down' (you'll learn that you need to go 'up' in order to sit 'down'!) are used to explore the value of inhibition and direction in making change in a fundamental pattern of movement. Lying down will now be a smaller part of the lesson time. Other basic procedures using the legs, arms and jaw – without disturbing the primary control – are gradually introduced. Detailed application of the Technique to the practicalities of living can then be tackled.

At some point the initial feeling of optimism may wear off as you reach your first learning plateau. Obvious improvement is set against what appears to be a huge amount of further work to be done. 'Alexander's gloom' has struck! This is the time to be philosophical and take a broader perspective. As Alexander said, 'It has taken us years to get wrong: we try to get right in an instant'.

Sometimes there is the thorny issue of whether a pupil should avoid a particular activity altogether until there is substantial improvement in his general condition or whether changes can be made while the habitual activity is modified. This is a matter for discussion with your teacher and involves a judgement based on your particular circumstances. For instance, if there appears to be a 'repetitive strain injury', how much damage has been caused? What are the pressures on you to continue the activity? How willing are you to approach it in a totally new way?

What is covered in lessons will vary from teacher to teacher. Teachers' *styles* of teaching may differ greatly and one approach may suit you more than others. You may be fortunate to have a range of teachers in your locality; the next section attempts

to outline some of the possible differences so that you can make
a more informed choice.

TEACHING STYLES

You may know the fable about the blind men who, each feeling
a different part of an elephant, came to somewhat different
conclusions about what the animal looked like. The elephant we
are concerned with is Alexander! Alexander trained one
generation of teachers, many of whom are no longer with us and
who interpreted his teaching *in their own ways*. The transmission
of his teaching is now entrusted to a second generation, and
increasingly to a third, far removed from the founder.
Differences of interpretation that have arisen are arguably only
differences of emphasis. But how recognizable is the elephant?
While some fear that the core of Alexander's original teaching
is in danger of being diluted, distorted and lost, others believe
that the way the Technique is taught should be radically
changed. Nowadays, in trying to identify some of the differences
it is not simply a question of which training a teacher has
received: a process of cross-fertilization has gone on and a mix
of styles has emerged.

The Operational Ideas

Lessons should contain the central intellectual and experiential
elements of the Technique. These are: inhibition and direction-
sending to the primary control as well as certain procedures that
will help you gain an understanding of how the operational ideas
apply to basic movement patterns. Some teachers will put more
emphasis on inhibition whereas others will stress the prime
importance of direction-sending. A proper balance needs to be
struck.

One result of the diversification of teacher training seems to
be that not all teachers understand the primary control in the
same way. What, exactly, is meant by the directions 'head
forward and up in relation to the back lengthening and
widening'? Alexander explained the directions to be given to the
primary control in *negative* terms, saying they were meant to

prevent the neck stiffening, the head pulling back and down and the back shortening and narrowing. So far, attempts to define the primary control – which can be clearly experienced subjectively – in an objective and measurable way, have been unsuccessful.

Is there any way of resolving this difficulty? Is it possible to pin down the dynamic and living nature of this central organizing principle? If what Alexander wrote is not conclusive, perhaps we could examine the tantalizingly short and poor-quality film record of him at work, made in the late 1940s – and now available on video (from STAT Books; see the Further Reading section) – to see what he *actually did*. What strikes me about the film is that Alexander clearly produces, in the people he is shown working with, what he called 'antagonistic muscular pulls' (one of the most gifted teachers Alexander trained, Patrick Macdonald, called this 'opposition'), whereby the back stays back in relation to the head – the spine lengthening – throughout all movement.

Manual Skill

Apart from *what* is being taught, there are naturally variations in teachers' levels of skill in conveying in practice *how* the primary control should work. Some training schools in trying to give weight to other aspects of teaching the Technique may underplay the importance of manipulative skills. As Alexander and others frequently pointed out, this brings the danger that verbal descriptions may be misunderstood. Words can only point to the thing described – they are not the thing itself. Conversely, relying too much on the teacher's hands brings the opposite danger – that the pupil may be less inclined to think for himself and not be able to make sufficient connection to the Technique in his life.

And so the two ingredients – hands-on experience and verbal directions – need to be linked clearly. The temptation to rely on vague images rather than the clear and concrete directions that Alexander devised should be avoided.

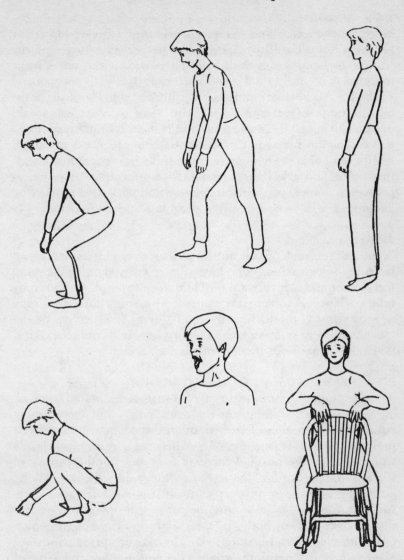

Figure 7: Procedures used to improve co-ordinated use of key parts of the body

Basic Procedures

Some teachers employ a fairly limited range of procedures. For instance not all will teach the 'monkey' in two stages or the 'lunge' or hands on a chair-rail or the whispered 'ah' – basic patterns of co-ordination involving, respectively, the proper use of the legs in bending and weight transfer, the use of the arms and of the jaw (see Figure 7). If this were the case you would not be getting all the basic tools you'd need to put Alexander's principles into practice. Furthermore, some teachers are more willing and able to demonstrate the links between Alexander's principles and procedures and their application to practical problems. Unless you can get help with making these links, the Technique will be of less value than it could be.

Working on Yourself

Some teachers prefer to say little in lessons; change is left to happen by itself. Such teachers often have very sensitive hands; the pupil feels better and a certain amount of release takes place. This may relieve whatever problem is presented. Also, some pupils naturally progress much more quickly than others, irrespective of the teacher. However, if you are not shown how to 'think in activity' you may remain dependent on such a teacher.

WHY LESSONS ARE NOT ALWAYS SUCCESSFUL

The Alexander Technique is not, of course, a method of *treatment*. To work properly it requires the conscious – and increasingly equal – participation of both pupil and teacher. The teacher's main responsibility is to take care of his own co-ordination while working with the pupil. When he asks the pupil to think of freeing the neck, the teacher – at the same time – will be attending to his own primary control: it is not a matter of one who has 'arrived' complacently dispensing received knowledge: the teacher's own body is the instrument through which anything meaningful is imparted. There needs to be a meeting place in lessons, therefore, where a deepening understanding of what the pupil may be doing to interfere with his own body use can be forged.

The Teacher's Responsibility

Occasionally lessons are started and then peter out because the teacher's manner appears – or even *is* – patronizing. 'It will all become clear to you one day, my dear' is infuriating if you need at least *something* to get your teeth into. It's true that no teacher will inform a pupil at his first lesson of all that trained eyes and hands can tell: to do so would be to burden him with detailed knowledge whose full significance at that stage could not possibly be understood and which might be quite dispiriting. There is a balance to be struck in the amount of information given. My preference is to err towards giving too much information and to encourage my pupils to experiment freely; their growing autonomy is what I understand to be the purpose of the Technique.

What should be the role of the teacher? He needs a certain authority that comes from his experience of having travelled further in a journey which, at first, may seem uncertain and confusing to the pupil. If the teacher is adaptable, he will be able to relate the Technique to a range of individual needs.

Another, less common reason for failure is that the co-ordination of the pupil may be so poor that it taxes the teacher's manual skills. In this case the pupil should be referred to a more skilled colleague as soon as possible, before any feelings of discouragement have time to set in.

The Pupil's Task

Our inclination is to do what gives us immediate pleasure or avoids pain, regardless of the consequences. It is easy to think of our health as someone else's responsibility. People sometimes delay starting Alexander lessons or fail to continue to work on themselves with the excuses of lack of time, too much stress, too little money or being too old – among others. While there is often some validity in these justifications, it is perhaps more true that fundamental change is uncomfortable. And some people seem to be so out of touch with their bodies that it can be especially hard for them to make any kind of connection.

Finally, a pupil's misuse may only be a small part of a

constellation of contributing causes which may be outside his control. In this case the Technique's effectiveness in relieving a certain condition is bound to be limited. If there has been spinal surgery or a major accident or injury or the pupil is older, or there is a condition like muscular sclerosis where there may well be irreversible damage, the Technique can have an important part to play in slowing down further deterioration. And to the extent that pupils learn more about themselves and how they function, lessons may give additional benefits.

In the final analysis, the most important aspect of learning is to become your own teacher. This does not, of course, exclude seeking out opportunities for working with teachers who have gone deeply into the Technique over the years. The process is life-long and challenging, but you can reap great benefits.

Some people may wish to go a stage further – to take a teacher-training course (see Appendix A: Training to Teach the Alexander Technique).

Chapter 6

The Technique and
the Healing Arts

F. M. Alexander had an insight into the unity of mind and body long before alternative forms of medicine became more generally accepted. His operational ideas are still complete and unassailable nearly 40 years after his death. No one has challenged fundamentally the accuracy or cogency of his main observations nor the validity of the conclusions he drew about how we can improve the 'use of the self'. The Technique stands on its own, largely separate from wave after wave of methods of relaxation, exercise and meditation, popular psychologies, burgeoning alternative/complementary therapies and the hegemony of orthodox medicine.

What is the path of healing and the role of self-help? The Technique has been described as a 'pre-technique': that is, it can help you to help yourself do anything you want to do. It gives you a yardstick by which you can judge your standard of co-ordination and how your activities may be affecting your health and well-being. This may lead to uncomfortable revelations about many things we take for granted; it can challenge the assumptions on which many of our attempts to help ourselves – or get help – have been based.

Let me give you an example from my own experience. I used to be a fitness fiend. I couldn't understand why, when I first began taking Alexander lessons, my teacher would ask me what I was doing between lessons to undermine her work with me. I prided myself on my fitness and it took some time before I began to *sense* how much I was harming myself thrashing a ball around the squash court or doing my yoga stretches.

In this chapter I will try to place the Alexander Technique in a wider context. To suit your particular needs you will need not only to have a clear understanding of what the Technique *is*, but also of what it is *not* and how it differs from other approaches. I have attempted to compare the Technique with those methods with which it might be confused and those with which it might in some way conflict.

To start with, what the Technique is *not*: similar to yoga; an expensive form of relaxation; of no benefit if you are in acute pain; incompatible with osteopathy; primarily a physical therapy. Can you mix the Alexander Technique with other disciplines? As a pre-technique it can certainly help you assess the merits and possible disadvantages of other approaches.

Manipulative Methods

Osteopathy and *chiropractic* are concerned with how structural problems, especially those of the spine, can disrupt body functioning. The Alexander Technique can complement these methods in that changes in body use will affect bodily structure and hence functioning. The beneficial effects of osteopathic/ chiropractic manipulation are also more likely to be maintained with the improved body use the Technique can bring. Furthermore, the osteopath's or chiropractor's task is made easier if the patient is more 'relaxed'. (A small number of Alexander teachers are also trained in manipulation, although they will not usually give a 'mixed' session.) There is no need to wait until you are 'well' before starting Alexander lessons – you can use it to support manipulative treatment – although there can be the problem that it may be difficult to know what is contributing the most to any improvement.

The professional relationship between osteopaths/ chiropractors and Alexander teachers has not always been as co-operative as it might be: many people consulting the osteopath/chiropractor expect to be 'fixed up' quickly. The practitioner may be drawn into symptomatic treatment which does not get to the root of the problem. Some practitioners may have an interest in 'repeat orders' – whereas Alexander work should *reduce* the need for manipulation by preventing problems or by speeding rehabilitation.

Here are some conditions for which an osteopath/chiropractor could consider referring a patient for lessons in the Alexander Technique:

- stress-related, psychosomatic disorders in tense individuals
- obvious malcoordination and poor posture; problems with balance
- nerve/muscle/bone problems
- developmental problems, e.g., scoliosis
- work-related conditions, e.g., 'repetitive strain injuries', back pain
- *recurrent* problems

Two questions the practitioner should keep in mind: 'Is the patient's condition mainly due to poor body use?' and, 'Is the patient motivated to help himself?' By putting these questions and applying the above criteria, patients who would benefit from Alexander lessons might be referred more appropriately.

Some Alexander teachers have reservations about the value of manipulation. The theory is that when the overall pattern of body use is improved through Alexander lessons, specific problems will be sorted out in the process, but if problems are treated in isolation – as may be the case with manipulative techniques – you may be creating further difficulties. It has also been claimed that manipulation itself can upset co-ordination (there is some evidence for this with less skilled manipulation) and that therefore Alexander work may be undermined. The counter-argument, of course, is that certain problems can take a considerable amount of time to clear up – if ever – if co-ordination is addressed alone. Such problems may benefit from the additional skills of an experienced osteopathic/chiropractic practitioner. I hope that there will be more informed contact between osteopaths/chiropractors and Alexander teachers and a better appreciation of the contributions each can make – this can only be of benefit.

MASSAGE, SHIATSU AND ROLFING AND ITS DERIVATIVES

The less deep forms of massage (such as *Swedish* and *aromatherapy* massages) can be very pleasant and can produce a certain amount of release of tension *at the time of treatment*. They make the patient aware of some excessive tension and some people find that this helps them open up to feelings that may be 'trapped' in their bodies. However, the limitation of these (and all) forms of massage is that the patient is passive; a course of treatment may not address the underlying causes. Although you may feel more relaxed and revitalized during and immediately after treatment, no essential change will have taken place in body use and you are likely to return to the lifestyle that created the problem in the first place. Also, hard as it may be to believe, *too much* relaxation may have been produced during the treatment.

The stated aim of *Shiatsu* and *acupressure* (derived from Oriental medicine), as well as of *reflexology*, is to influence the subtle energy channels that are said to exist in the body. Thus these methods are in no essential conflict with the Technique. Indeed, to the extent that these and other 'energy-balancing' therapies work, the Alexander technique may enhance a person's ability to maintain improvement.

The assumptions underlying *Rolfing* (Ida Rolf's method) and its derivatives, e.g. Heller, Postural Integration and others, do seem to have a certain incompatibility with those of the Alexander Technique. Rolfing stresses the need for structural realignment, in which parts of the body are to be 're-stacked' on top of other parts. Compare this with the Alexander model – more a suspension of parts from above than any kind of stacking. Rolfing massage is very deep and is often accompanied by considerable emotional release. These emotional changes are not sought directly in Alexander work although they may occur none the less, usually in an unforced way, as part of the gradual transformation of one's physical co-ordination. A course of Rolfing is often followed by an attempt to 're-pattern' movement. From the Alexander point of view, it is difficult to see how this can be truly successful unless the issue of faulty kinaesthesia – underlying malcoordination – is addressed.

Finally, all the practitioners mentioned so far – in fact all physical therapists – could benefit greatly from Alexander work because of the stresses of the awkward positions they themselves often adopt while working on patients.

Relaxation Techniques

Alexander held that relaxation techniques are potentially harmful because they often lead to a generalized loss of muscle tone. Moreover, these techniques do little to help the patient in stressful situations because he has not acquired the skills of flexible and appropriate distribution of muscle tension needed for each activity. All the following widely-known methods were developed by doctors.

Progressive Relaxation (outlined by Jacobson in 1929) has you tense and then relax in sequence muscle groups throughout the body while sitting, back supported, or lying down (no support for the head is advocated). This is supposed to increase your awareness of tension and how you can release it. However, while you will certainly notice a difference between being tense and relaxed, there is evidence that the level of tension *after* you perform this procedure is actually *higher* than beforehand. Incomplete release may have taken place, and the more you tense yourself the more tolerant and unaware you become of excessive tension.

Benson's *Relaxation Method*, derived from Transcendental Meditation, involves repeating a 'mantra' or word, twice a day, usually in a sitting position. If you want to make a regular practice of meditation, Alexander lessons can help you cope better with the tendency of the body to become stiff and heavy from prolonged sitting still.

Autogenic Training, devised by Schulz, is a method of auto-suggestion. F. M. Alexander had two main reservations about this kind of approach. First of all, the messages given (such as, 'my arm feels heavy') – if effective – will almost certainly induce a pulling down *throughout* the body. Secondly, attempts made to influence the autonomic/involuntary nervous system *directly* (such as 'my heart beat feels calm') are most undesirable, according to Alexander. The autonomic system has its own inherent 'wisdom' and should not be tampered with. Alexander's 'thinking in activity' can reduce the impact of stress. By releasing the neck muscles and maintaining a proper, balanced muscle tone throughout the body the autonomic nervous system naturally and spontaneously tends to rebalance itself.

Exercise and Movement

Alexander made some very cogent observations about the methods of physical culture and deep-breathing exercises that were becoming popular in his day. He noted that when you give ten people the same exercise to do, it will be done in ten idiosyncratic ways. The pattern of movement will reflect a person's *idea* of how the movement should be performed, which will be based on unreliable kinaesthesia. The faster and more frequently the movement is performed, the more faulty patterns of use will become consolidated and exaggerated. *No* form of exercise is safe, contrary to what anyone peddling the latest fitness craze will claim. (Notice the let-out clause in small print: consult your doctor first. However, he may be as little aware as most of us of the unreliability of our kinaesthetic sense.)

The only exception to these reservations about all forms of exercise applies to the very few individuals whose kinaesthesia is registering accurately – and they don't need to do special exercises.

SUPPLENESS

Hatha Yoga claims to be the ideal way of cultivating a healthy body through the practice of certain postures and breathing exercises. Many of the postures demand quite exceptional suppleness; for someone who is already supple, yoga can be very enjoyable. There is, however, a serious risk of producing hypermobility in certain joints. It is said that yoga postures should not be considered as ends in themselves, but as means whereby the energies in the body can be helped to flow; and that, therefore, the process of attempting a posture is more important than achieving or holding it. Unfortunately, the less supple members of a yoga class, even though exhorted by the teacher not to force or overexert themselves – but only too aware of the litheness of others – often subtly and obliviously do just that. And there is an additional problem: when parts of the body stiffen, adjacent parts become abnormally mobile. It is these parts that will tend to move when you try to free the stiffer ones (compare this to the manipulative therapy technique of mobilizing stiff joints by splinting looser ones).

Most of us, prior to Alexander work, have little conscious knowledge of everyday movements, of how we are standing, sitting or lying down *before* we attempt a yoga position. Even the so-called 'relaxation' pose – lying on the back, head falling back down towards the floor, arms close to the sides, palms turned up – encourages precisely the pattern of misuse that Alexander discovered was the root cause of his vocal trouble and which is such a problem for most of us. You may, therefore, find that there is some conflict between yoga and the Alexander principles; as a pre-technique, however, the Alexander Technique can certainly help you practise yoga in the most effective, least harmful way.

There is a good case for basic *stretching* movements, to help maintain flexibility as we get older; and currently there is a lot of interest in stretching as a means of preventing injuries, especially for athletes and sportspeople. What, though, is being advocated? Which joints will be involved and how is the stretch to be made? Very few of us know how to stretch without creating unnecessary tension. Bouncing into a stretch – which is usually what happens in aerobics classes – can be especially harmful and should be avoided. This is one advantage of yoga, where you go slowly into a stretch and sustain it, endeavouring to release into the stretch. Furthermore, if you exercise vigorously you boost your blood levels of endorphins (morphine-related chemicals produced in the body). This carries the danger of numbing any pain signals your brain might be receiving. It is possible to get hooked on the 'high' of vigorous exercise.

The final point is this: *unless you really know what you are doing, you are likely to be binding up the key joints – the head-neck and hip joints – on whose freedom the natural suppleness of the rest of your body depends.* The freedom of these joints depends on a *release* into length and a certain 'opposition' of adjacent parts of the body. This opposition is very difficult to find unless you have experienced it repeatedly in Alexander lessons.

STAMINA

It is commonly held that unless you exercise vigorously at least three times a week, boosting your pulse rate, you cannot be creating optimum health. But what are most people doing in the attempt to improve their cardiovascular system? They are increasing muscle tension unduly throughout their bodies and their hearts are being forced to work considerably harder than they should.

Your body and its organs have a finite lifespan. You may actually be *shortening* your life as well as causing damage to other parts of your body – particularly your joints – by overexercise. The fixing of your lowermost, floating ribs as your chest lifts and your lower back hollows – which occurs when most people exercise hard, accompanied by sucking in air – encourages harmful breathing habits: there will be an overemphasis on expansion of the upper chest rather than on expansion of the lower thorax. Add to the equation extra stress on your joints – even with 'low-impact' aerobics – and the demonstrable disadvantages of aerobic exercise may outweigh the benefits. Perhaps a more sensible beginning to healthy living would be to ask, 'How can I avoid wasting my energies in all my daily activities?'

STRENGTH/TONING

Here we are concerned with the commonly-held idea that you should do something special to exercise particular muscle groups. If you are not clear enough about how the body works as a whole, you run the risk of creating all sorts of imbalances.

The fitness equipment now available, designed for working out selected muscle groups, is very sophisticated. But if you observe what actually happens in the gym (whatever the initial training offered by the instructors), you will see very few people using the equipment as intended. Most people, especially in the group context, inevitably get into an 'end-gaining' mode. They load up the weights and recruit muscles all over the body – and especially neck muscles – when the focus should be on the appropriate use of specific muscle groups. Nor does all this effort necessarily make them stronger: the amount of power a person can command has little to do with brute force and more to do with technique and co-ordination.

In summary, then, the emphasis on developing suppleness, stamina, strength or speed in isolation neglects *co-ordination*, the underpinning factor in the effectiveness and efficiency with which the body works as a whole – with the mind. Exercise that most of us can enjoy and which, to a large degree can, if reasonably well done, compensate for a sedentary lifestyle includes walking, cycling, some forms of folk-dancing, swimming and T'ai Chi.

T'ai Chi
T'ai Chi is the softest martial art from China. As usually practised in the West – at a basic level – its health aspects are primary. The popular Yang-style 'form' consists of slow, flowing, circular movements that are practised daily and take between 5 and 20 minutes to perform. The idea is to move from your body's centre of gravity (the *tan t'ien*, just below the navel – equivalent to the Japanese *hara*). In the 'classic' T'ai Chi texts there is a description of the essential features of the form. The first three appear to be a formulation of Alexander's primary control. In most of the movements (others can be modified) there is no need to compromise the primary control at all. All the major joints are moved gently through a wide range of movement. The legs recover much of their power and suppleness. The mental effects are clear: if you let your attention wander at all, you soon start to wobble and lose your balance.

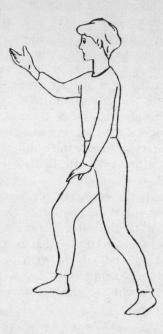

Figure 8: T'ai Chi can promote health and well-being. It allows the proper use of the primary control to co-ordinate slow, flowing movement

How different from slumping over an exercise cycle, pumping away – some people even try to read whilst exercising as if mind and body are separate!

I suspect that if Alexander were alive today and observed T'ai Chi in action, his reservations about it would be much more muted than for exercise in general.

T'ai Chi is suitable for most people and especially for older people because of its slowness and gentleness. Part of its appeal lies in the fascination of constantly refining the quality of movement. Unlike most exercise programs you are not likely to get bored – it is far too challenging. You may at times feel daunted by the extent of learning that there is to do, but any improvement is worthwhile and can be built upon.

Students and teachers of T'ai Chi can benefit from a working knowledge of Alexander's principles of inhibition, direction and the problem of faulty kinaesthesia. Equally, students of the Alexander Technique who decide to learn T'ai Chi will have their understanding of Alexander's principles challenged and perhaps enriched: T'ai Chi is an ideal medium for applying Alexander principles to movement.

Feldenkrais Method

Feldenkrais was a physicist and black belt in judo who, owing to a serious knee problem which doctors told him would require the use of a walking stick, researched widely in the biological sciences, took lessons in the Alexander Technique and then developed his own method. It has two aspects: *Functional Integration* – individual therapeutic work involving touch – and *Awareness through Movement* – taught in group settings.

A Feldenkrais teacher gives a bare description of a movement to be explored without any suggestion that there is a 'right' way to do it. The accent is on awareness and learning to move *slowly* in effortless ways. Complex movement patterns are broken down into their components and then re-integrated so that new possibilities of movement can be discovered.

This method is a creative exploration into the basics of how we move. Feldenkrais was indebted to Alexander for many of his ideas. My impression is that there is a considerable amount of value in Feldenkrais work, especially if you have a good grounding in the Technique. From what I have seen, the process of learning looks more uncertain if you haven't had prior Alexander work because there is no emphasis on the importance of the primary control and the role of direction-giving. So, although Feldenkrais and Alexander work are based on different premises, each can contribute to the other.

Psychotherapies

A major limitation of the Technique is that it does not address the significance of our emotional and spiritual sides: Alexander did not ask *why* but in *what way* his striving to project his voice affected his co-ordination. His quest led him to link his manner of use with *intention* rather than emotional complexes. He was rather dismissive of psychoanalysis; he felt it had no working model of the mind/body unit as the vehicle for change. (This, of course, is not true of later developments such as bioenergetics and the humanistic psychotherapies, which are very body-orientated.)

The physical changes that take place during Alexander lessons, although unforced, are often very profound. If I am no longer entirely my bundle of physical attitudes and postures, with which I was previously identified, who am I? For some people the psychological adjustments are integrated spontaneously with the physical ones; for others there may be the welling up of quite deep emotions. If this happens and your teacher seems disconcerted, do not worry! That is his problem, not yours. Perhaps you should change teachers if you feel uncomfortable about continuing. Sometimes counselling or psychotherapy can be of benefit at such a time (your Alexander teacher may be able to refer you to someone).

The Alexander Technique can provide us with a very effective and efficient mental/physical 'machine' for everyday living. It has, however, little to say about what our lives should be and why some choices are more desirable than others. In the next chapter, we shall look at why taking the Alexander Technique on board may also involve reframing our life goals.

Chapter 7

Taking Charge of Your Life

What our lives are all about is not so much the search for meaning as the rapturous experience of being alive, according to Joseph Campbell, the great authority on the function of myth as an aid to self-understanding. [1]

Alexander had little to say about what our life purposes might be other than stressing the desirability of seeking more harmony of mind and body in all our daily actions. His image of 'true happiness' is the 'healthy child busily engaged in doing something which interests it.' Adults, argued Alexander, lose this as they experience a deterioration in body use and the accompanying feelings of irritability and stress. Disappointments can sap self-confidence. We get on with our lives, giving little conscious attention to the 'daily round' and, as physical decline sets in, less and less are we able to experience that rapture of being alive – part of which is the pleasure of doing simple things and the delight of the unexpected; and we may rely on rather exotic ways of gaining pleasure or comfort.

Stated like this, Alexander can sound rather puritanical (he probably was), but I think he has a point. Commenting on what was then a relatively new phenomenon – large numbers of people reaching 'retirement' for the first time and not being able to cope with it – Alexander's explanation was that patterns of behaviour can become so limited and fixed that adaptation to changing circumstances is very difficult. [2]

Ends and Means
Most people coming for Alexander lessons seek relief from a

variety of physical – and sometimes mental – symptoms. As they find out what they are doing that may be contributing to their difficulties, they begin to question whether they are employing the appropriate means to achieve the ends they seek. This investigation may need to go no further than discovering, for instance, how one's neck and back problems are created by working at a visual display unit all day long and how to prevent the problem by learning a more *active* way of sitting so that the proper length of the spine can be maintained (assisted, of course, by the relevant ergonomic adjustments).

Not infrequently, though, other issues may surface. A person might ask himself, 'How much longer do I want to work at a computer? Is there something else I would rather be doing? And where am I going with my life?' In short, the presenting problem may mask a larger underlying crisis in a person's life. A crisis, the Chinese believe, holds out not only the threat of danger but also its opposite – the opportunity for constructive change. How might you begin finding your way through such a crisis?

The discipline of the Alexander Technique requires some order in your daily life if you are to take it on board as a tool for life-long self-development.

Larry, a former actor, came for lessons after years of chronic back pain, only ever getting temporary relief - at best - from all the various practitioners he consulted.

His first Alexander lesson made it quite clear to him that his pain was caused almost entirely by his own tension patterns. After a course of lessons his pain had gone. However, he began to feel more and more concerned by all the powerful and conflicting emotions that began to surface. The possibility of counselling was raised but Larry found that the Technique could be applied to emotional reactions - that he could stay calm and centred under duress. He now had much more energy than he had experienced for a long time. He has now decided to follow a different career and is training to be a teacher. Even the demands of dealing with a class of children with learning disabilities have not lead to any return of his back problems and the Technique has helped him keep his head in confrontational situations.

The rest of this chapter touches on clarifying our ends and means. Remarkable overlap between the Alexander Technique and, among other methods, aspects of Gurdjieff's work on the self and that of Zen Buddhism have been noted[3]; but I shall try to put the Alexander Technique in a broader context (hopefully not inimical to Alexander's basic assumptions).

One starting point is that human nature is essentially purposeful and problem-solving and that our activities are more or less 'reasonable' whether or not we can define easily what those reasons are. We seem also to have a clear existential choice between living our lives at the mercy of things that happen to us or playing a large part in planning and creating our life's story. The orthodox religious view is that we are instruments of a greater destiny and that it is not our place to reason why. The alternative view is that it is we who create meaning or significance in our lives; and, notwithstanding how things may be in an afterlife, what should we make of our lives here on this Earth?

What's Important in Your Life?

Many commentators on the human condition have held that the overriding purpose in our lives is to find work that we love to do and to give a great deal of attention to achieving excellence at it – after all, most adults spend the largest chunk of their lives in employment. That is an enormous challenge in itself, but what about the conflicts that come with the need to find time for our loved ones as well? And what about the need for some leisure time for recreation, for self-development away from the demands of work and family? At certain times in life it is all too easy to feel completely 'boxed-in' with no time for a more balanced range of activities. One way to find a more creative balance is to take some of your scarce and valuable time to try to orientate yourself, to find out where you want to be going and to make realistic plans for change. The exercises in Richard Bolles' books on life/work planning[4] are excellent for this purpose – engagingly and humorously written and copiously illustrated.

You might want to take some time to set yourself some hypothetical challenges and see what comes to mind. A few examples are:

- Take a minute to list the five things that are most important to you at this point in your life.
- What would you do with your life if you had no financial limitations?
- What have you done in the past that has given you the most satisfaction and feelings of self-worth?
- What would you do with your life if you only had six months/one year/two years to live?
- If you wrote your own obituary, what would it say about you?

Taking time to explore these larger issues can be helpful in rekindling your energies for striking a better balance between family and friendship goals, career aspirations and personal development. At the same time we need to be reminded that our life goals need to take seed in the here and now – being clear about our immediate purposes, doing what needs to be done and accepting our feelings as they arise, however painful or disconcerting they sometimes may be.

Happiness as the Most Important Goal

According to Aristotle, we should guard against trying to maximize the contentment that we get from satisfying our immediate wants; instead we should seek happiness as an *ethical* state in a whole life well-lived. [5] This should be our ultimate end. We owe it to ourselves to live a good life and therefore *we should desire what is really good for us*. To do so we need to distinguish between the *apparent* goods that we may *want* and the *real* goods that we *need*. There is a clear parallel here with Alexander's indirect approach to achieving our ends: under the pressures of everyday life it is often easier to fall back on old patterns of response, even though we *know*, in our hearts, that they do not serve our long-term interests!

REAL GOODS AND HOW THEY ARE TO BE SOUGHT
What are these real goods that we need to be happy and live a good life? Aristotle says that we require health and well-being in abundance, a certain amount of material wealth for our physical needs and what he calls 'goods of the soul': the ability to exercise our reason (which we need in fullest measure), as well as friendship, pleasures of the mind (for instance, contemplating beauty) and the self-esteem and honour gained through 'right' action.

How are these goods to be sought? By making the best choices and decisions as opportunity presents. This will move us towards our ultimate goal of a good life. In time, we will be more habitually disposed to act in ways that are in our better interests. Alexander's 'thinking in activity' – inhibition and the need to attend to the proper means/whereby to accomplish our ends – therefore bears a similarity to Aristotle's 'practical' thinking.

The Alexander Technique and the Good Life
There are clearly many interesting points of contact between Aristotle's philosophy and Alexander's pragmatic approach. First of all, we find both advocating the use of reason and scientific method to solve problems. Secondly, both demonstrate a clear understanding of the relationship between means and ends. Thirdly, both put forward the idea that we need to exercise choice continually about the direction in which we want to go. And, finally, both recognize the importance of cultivating our health as part of living a good life.

So, taking stock of our situation can reaffirm the lasting value of the Alexander Technique as a means of improving the quality of the whole of our lives.

Appendix A

Training to Teach
the Alexander Technique

Some people undertake training not out of any prior strong motivation to teach but because they want the almost daily work practice in the Technique that a training course provides. This may appeal if you have severe difficulties and need intensive work for yourself, or you may be interested in the great opportunities that the Technique can offer you in the way of self-development.

In 1987 the UK's Society of Teachers of the Alexander Technique (STAT) carried out a survey of its members to find out about trends in teaching. Only a third of those who responded earned most of their income from teaching the Technique; the rest relied on other employment, on their partners or on private income. Unless you are training teachers yourself, if you expect to gain a substantial and secure income from teaching the Alexander Technique the message has to be: think again! With increasing numbers of people training, the supply of teachers appears to be outstripping demand, especially in the more desirable urban areas. On the other hand, teaching the Technique can provide an adequate income and flexible hours if you are interested in part-time work and/or in being self-employed.

Training courses normally last three years and involve 1600 hours' tuition. Attempts are underway to standardize training. There are at present 16 approved training courses in the UK, including six in London. Other approved training courses are available in the Netherlands (1), Australia, Denmark and France (2 each), Germany (3), Israel, Italy and Switzerland (5 each) and the US (6). For further information please send a stamped, addressed envelope to the Alexander Technique society in your country (see Useful Addresses).

References

Chapter 1
1. W. Barlow, *The Alexander Principle* (Arrow, 1990).
2. Letter to the *British Medical Journal*, 1, 1937, p. 1137.

Chapter 3
I am greatly indebted to the following sources about Alexander and his work, on which most of the information in this chapter is based:

W. H. M. Carrington, *On the Alexander Technique, in conversation with Sean Carey* (Sheldrake Press, 1986).
—— (ed.), *F. Matthias Alexander 1869 – 1955: A Biographical Outline* (Sheldrake Press, 1979).
F. P. Jones, *Body Awareness in Action: A Study of the Alexander Technique* (Schocken Books, 1988).
L. Westfeldt, *F. Matthias Alexander: the Man and His Work* (Centreline Press, 1986).

Chapter 4
1. F. P. Jones, *Body Awareness in Action: A Study of the Alexander Technique* (Schocken Books, 1988).
2. V. C. Abrahams, in D. Garlick (ed.), *Proprioception, Posture and Emotion* (University of New South Wales, 1982).
3. R. Soames and C. Stevens, cited in C. Stevens, *The Alexander Review*, 4, 1989, p. 181.
4. G. Tengwall, cited in J. Nicholls and S. Carey, *The Alexander Technique* (published by the authors, 1991).

5. B. Libet et al, 'Brain stimulation in the study of neuronal functions for conscious sensory experience', *Human Neurobiology*, 1, 1982, pp. 235 – 42.

6. ──, 'Unconscious cerebral initiative and the role of conscious will in voluntary action', *Behavioural and Brain Sciences*, 8, 1985, pp. 529 – 66.

7. F. Bojsen-Moller, R. Soames and C. Stevens, 'Influence of Initial Posture on the Sit to Stand Movement', *European Journal of Applied Physiology*, e58, 1989, pp. 687 – 92.

8. J. Basmajian, 'Conscious Control of Single Nerve Cells', *New Scientist*, 369, 1963, pp. 662–4.

9. D. Garlick, *The Lost Sixth Sense* (University of New South Wales, 1990).

10. *Ibid*

11. M. Nielsen, B. Christiensen and C. Stevens, cited in C. Stevens, *The Alexander Review*, 4, 1989, p. 181.

12. W. Barlow, *The Alexander Principle* (Arrow, 1990).

Chapter 6

1. The famous philosopher-sage, J. Krishnamurti, was reported to have damaged his neck through the practice of Iyengar yoga. He eventually switched to the gentler Desikachar yoga (see Ian Rawlinson's *Yoga for the West*).

Chapter 7

1. J. Campbell, *The Power of Myth* (Doubleday, 1989).

2. F. M. Alexander, *Constructive Conscious Control of the Individual* (Centreline Press, (1923), 1985; Part IV, 'Sensory appreciation in relation to happiness').

3. For an overview of the Technique in relation to depth psychology, bodywork and Eastern disciplines, see John Nicholl's 1986 Memorial Lecture, *The Alexander Technique in a Larger Context* (booklet available from STAT books – 20 London House, 266 Fulham Road, London SW10 9EL). This lecture also appears as an Appendix in John Nicholl's *The Alexander Technique* (also available from STAT books).

Glen Park's *The Art of Changing* (Ashgrove Press, 1989)

attempts to link the Technique to esoteric thought.

See P. Macdonald, *The Alexander Technique As I See It* (Rahula Books, 1989), among many other worthwhile things, for a reference to E. Herrigel, *Zen in the Art of Archery* (Routledge, 1953).

4. R. N. Bolles, *What Colour is Your Parachute?: A Practical Manual for Job-Hunters and Career-Changers* (Ten Speed Press, 1972).

Also see his *The Three Boxes of Life and How to Get out of Them: An introduction to Life/Work Planning* (Ten Speed Press, 1978).

5. I am greatly indebted to Mortimer Adler's admirably clear expositions of Aristotle's philosophy. See M. J. Adler, *Aristotle for Everybody: Difficult Thought Made Easy* (Macmillan, 1978). Also his *The Time of Our Lives* and *Ten Philosophical Mistakes* (both Macmillan, 1985).

Further Reading

Here is a highly selective list of books on the Alexander Technique. I have tried to include books that make an original contribution or that are authoritative sources of information. For a more comprehensive list of books and mail-order service in the UK, send a stamped, addressed envelope to STAT Books, 20 London House, 266 Fulham Road, London SW10 9EL.

Introductory Books
W. Barlow, *The Alexander Principle* (Arrow, 1990).

M. Gelb, *Body Learning: An Introduction to the Alexander Technique* (Aurum Press, 1987).

F. M. Alexander and His Technique
F. P. Jones, *Body Awareness in Action: A Study of the Alexander Technique* (Schocken Books, 1988).

L. Westfeldt, *F. Matthias Alexander: The Man and His Work* (Centreline Press, 1986).

Alexander's Writings
E. Maisel (ed.), *Alexander Technique – the Essential Writings of F. Matthias Alexander* (Thames and Hudson, 1989).

Contains, among other key passages, the first chapter of *The Use of the Self*, 'The Evolution of the Technique' ('The Australian Story').

Working on Yourself/Applying the Technique to Your Life

A. and J. Drake and I. Machover, *The Alexander Birth Guide* (Robinson, 1993).

J. Drake, *Body Know-How: A Practical Guide to the Use of the Alexander Technique in Everyday Life* (Thorsons, 1991).

J. Gray, *Your Guide to the Alexander Technique* (Gollancz, 1990).

Useful Addresses

The following will provide lists of teachers who have completed the three-year approved training course (please send a stamped addressed envelope):

UK
The Society of Teachers of the Alexander Technique (STAT)
20 London House
266 Fulham Rd
London SW10 9EL
Tel: 071 – 351 0828

Australia
Australian Society of Teachers of the Alexander Technique (AUSTAT)
PO Box 529
Milson's Point
NSW 2061

Canada
Canadian Society of Teachers of the Alexander Technique (CANSTAT)
Box 502
Station E
Montreal
Quebec H2T 3A9
Tel: (514) 598 – 8879

Denmark
Danish Society of Teachers of the Alexander Technique (DFLAT)
c/o Mary McGovern
Sandhojen 18
DK-2720 Vanlose
Tel: 31 741366

Germany
German Society of Teachers of the Alexander Technique (GLAT)
Postfach 5312
7800 Freiburg
Tel: 0761 475995

Israel
Israeli Society of Teachers of the Alexander Technique (ISTAT)
c/o Nelken
26 Radak Street
Jerusalem
Tel: 02 660683

The Netherlands
The Netherlands Society of Teachers of the Alexander Technique
Max Havelaarlaan 80
1183 H N Amstelveen
Tel: 020 439052

South Africa
South African Society of Teachers of the Alexander Technique (SASTAT)
35 Thornhill Rd
Rondebosch 7700
Tel: 021 686 8454

Switzerland
Swiss Society of Teachers of the Alexander Technique (SVLAT)
Postfach
CH-8032
Zurich

USA
North American Society of Teachers of the Alexander Technique
PO Box 3992
Champaign, IL
61826-3992
Tel: (217) 359 - 3529

There are also qualified teachers in Austria, Belgium, Brazil, Colombia, Eire, Finland, France, Hong Kong, Iceland, Italy, Japan, Luxemburg, Malaysia, Mexico, New Zealand, Norway, Pakistan, Poland, Spain and Sweden; and more teachers are being trained all the time. You can find out about teachers not represented by a national body through the UK Society of Teachers of the Alexander Technique (address and telephone number above).

Index